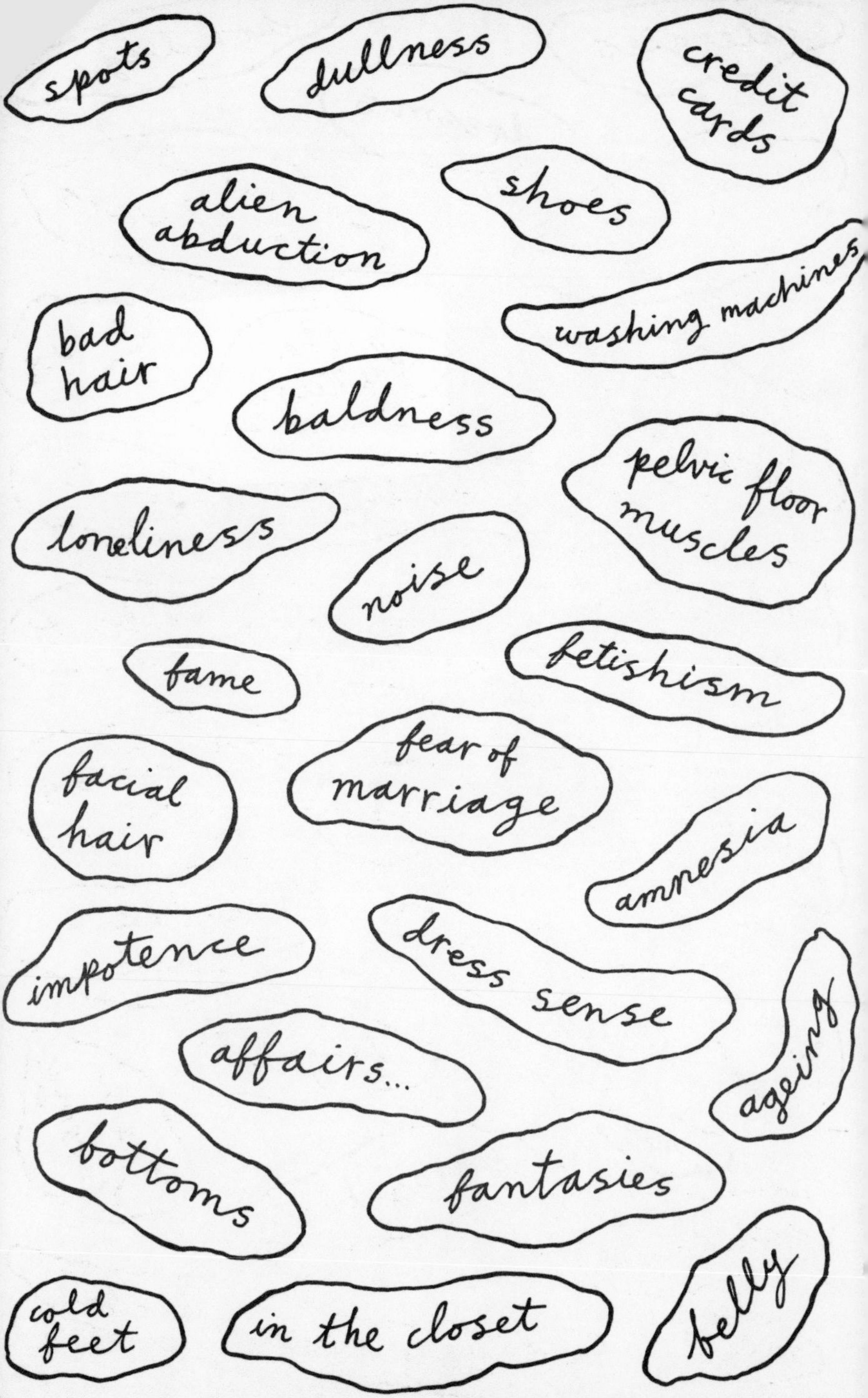

spots

dullness

credit cards

alien abduction

shoes

washing machines

bad hair

baldness

pelvic floor muscles

loneliness

noise

fame

fetishism

facial hair

fear of marriage

amnesia

impotence

dress sense

affairs...

ageing

bottoms

fantasies

cold feet

in the closet

belly

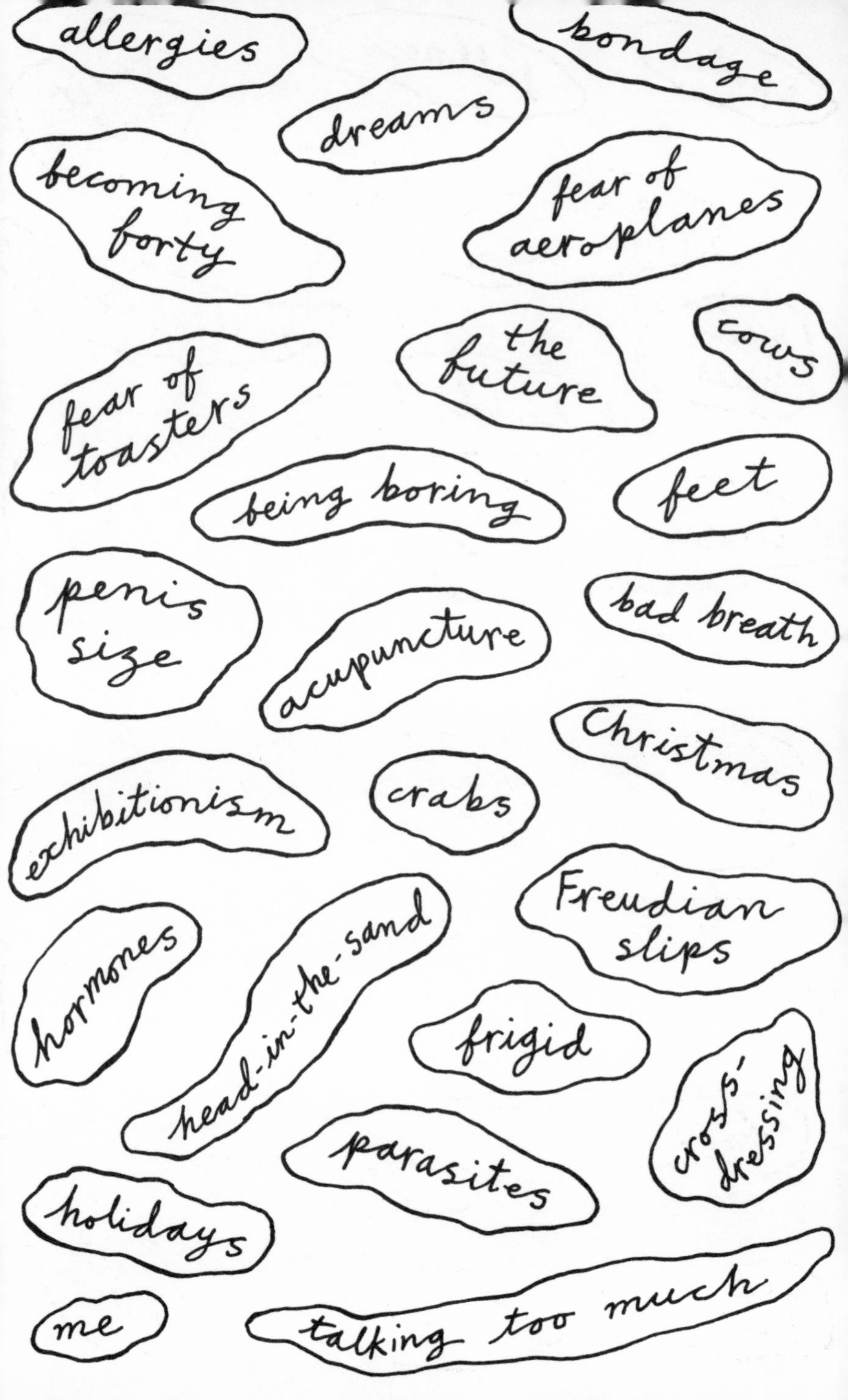

allergies

bondage

dreams

becoming forty

fear of aeroplanes

the future

cows

fear of toasters

being boring

feet

penis size

acupuncture

bad breath

Christmas

exhibitionism

crabs

Freudian slips

hormones

head-in-the-sand

frigid

cross' dressing

holidays

parasites

me

talking too much

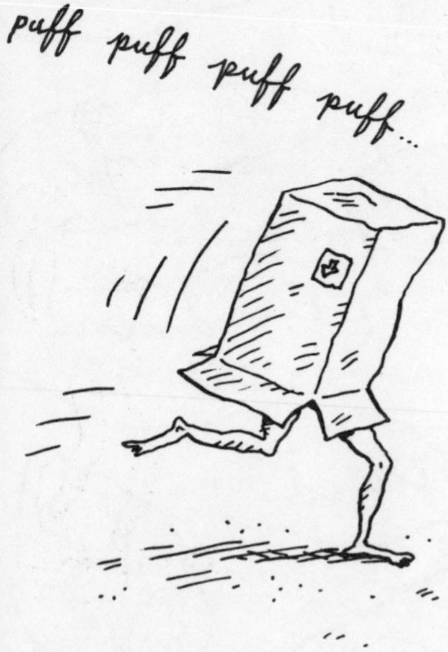
puff puff puff puff...

## DISCLAIMER

Buying, or being given, this book DOES NOT in ANY WAY infer (or imply) that <u>YOU</u> suffer from any, some or even EVERY problem listed within. This book is of curiosity value only. So why not, purely out of curiosity, turn to IN DENIAL (page 94).

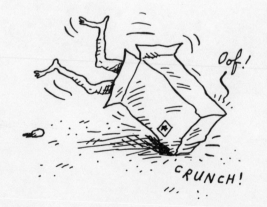

Oof!

CRUNCH!

# ENCYCLOPEDIA OF PERSONAL PROBLEMS

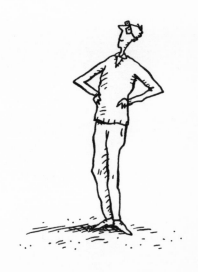

# Steven Appleby's ENCYCLOPEDIA of PERSONAL PROBLEMS

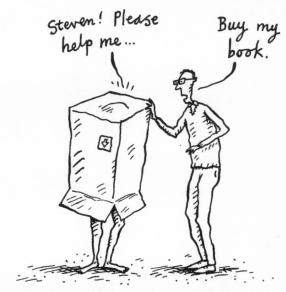

BY STEVEN APPLEBY
AND A. FRIEND

BLOOMSBURY

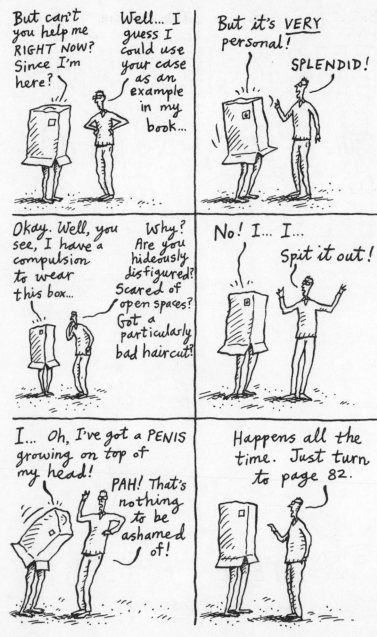

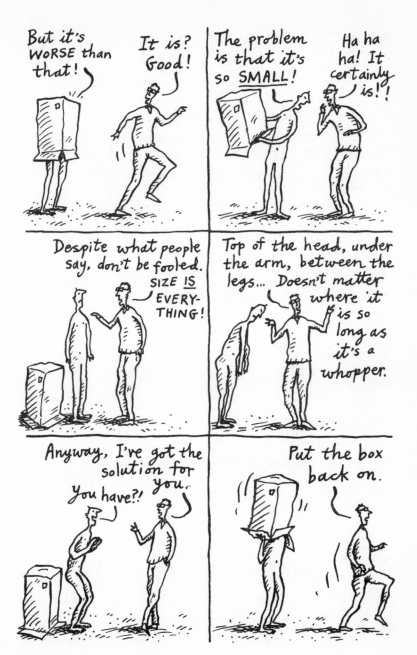

11

MANY THANKS TO:
Jonny Boatfield, Pete Bishop, Karen Brown,
Liz Calder, Kasper de Graaf, Janny Kent,
LWW, George Mole, Polly Napper, Nicola
Sherring, Mary Tomlinson, Simon Thomas,
Jonny White, everyone at Bloomsbury & all my
friends without whose personal problems
this book would not have been possible.

MANY OF THE IDEAS AND THEMES IN THIS
BOOK HAVE BEEN DEVELOPED FROM DRAWINGS
WHICH FIRST APPEARED IN: The Guardian,
The Sunday Telegraph, Harpers & Queen, Junior,
Company, The Erotic Review and The New
York Times.

SPECIAL THANKS TO: A. Friend (grudgingly...)

BLOOMSBURY PUBLISHING PLC
38 SOHO SQUARE, LONDON W1D 3HB

ISBN 0 7475 5307 6

PRINTED IN GREAT BRITAIN BY OMNIA BOOKS LTD
10 9 8 7 6 5 4 3 2 1

Dear reader,

May I humbly point out that in YOUR interest I have _personally_ tested every single problem covered by this book. Or my friend has. A problem shared is a problem halved. Or doubled. I forget which, but I'm sure it helps.

I hope you get better soon...

Your author,

Steven Appleby

June 21· 2000.

# HOW TO USE THIS UP-TO-THE-MINUTE REFERENCE SYSTEM

We like to think of this book as a convenient, hand-held website which you can consult without needing an expensive computer or phone line! Simply activate your SEARCH ENGINE (BRAIN) by visualising the problem you want information about (for example, CHILDREN) in your DIALOGUE BOX (MIND'S EYE). Next, use your INTERFACE (HANDS) to flip through the pages (ingeniously ordered using an alphabetical filing system) until you locate the subject you first thought of. Now, utilise your eyes to transfer data from the page into your mind. Congratulations! The valuable information you requested is now stored in your memory bank to be accessed when needed in order to improve your life.

# ETYMOLOGY

You'll find INSECTS under INSECTS!
This straight-talking book has
no use for long and difficult
words which noone understands!

# ABBREVIATIONS

There ARE no abbreviations used
in this work! The author and
publisher don't believe in cutting
corners or leaving things out.
This book brings you everything
IN FULL!

## ABDUCTION (BY ALIENS) ~ far more common than people think. In fact, most of us have been abducted many times. I know I have. Look out for unexplained scars:

BEFORE ~          AFTER ~

Forgetting names, faces and phone numbers is a sign that your brain has been removed and experimented on.

See also: AMNESIA, & below.

## ABSENT-MINDEDNESS

~ Usually comes on following ALIEN ABDUCTION. I certainly couldn't remember a thing after mine. Walking into a room and thinking: "What on earth did I come in here for?" is a sure sign that you've just been abducted, dissected and returned with your memory wiped clean.

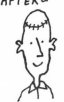

Is this my room?

See also: DELUDING YOURSELF (though I'm not!).

## ABSTINENCE ~ the masochistic decision to deny yourself something you want such as food or sex. If you must practise ABSTINENCE my tip is to abstain from something you DON'T like, such as being run down by a lawnmower, or sticking your fingers into a toaster.

Abstaining from watching Saturday night TV is easy!

See also: DIETING.

# A

## ACHES & PAINS ~
This description is a bit too general to be of much use. Where are the aches? In your head? Arm? Tummy? Leg? Groin? Look up something more specific next time.

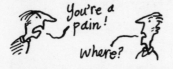

## SOME USEFUL ACUPUNCTURE POINTS:
### i - EAR.
OUCH!

### ii - BOTTOM.
Yow!

### iii - WILLY.
No!! Keep away!

It's for your own good!

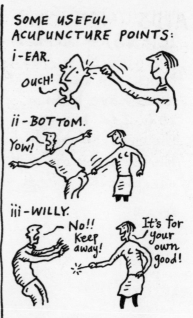

## ACNE ~ See SPOTS
(Not SEEING SPOTS. That's a different problem).

## ACUPUNCTURE ~
A form of voodoo in which pins are stuck directly into the person you want to harm. Obviously much more effective than using a wax effigy.

ow! What did you do that for?!!

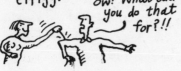

## ADDICTION ~ the
inability to ABSTAIN.

## AFFAIR ~ What
men and women do if they think they can get away with it. An affair starts out as uncomplicated sex, then quickly becomes very complicated indeed.

See also: DECEIT; DIVORCE; MURDER; GUILT; DESPAIR; DEPRESSION & FUN.

18

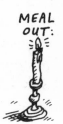

**AIDS (MARITAL)** ~ Here are a selection of useful sex aids which can help keep a marriage on course:

FLOWERS:

CHOCOLATES:

TICKETS TO THE THEATRE:

MEAL OUT:

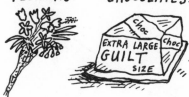

NEW SHOES:

PERFUME:

FLIGHT TO PARIS:

FACIAL:

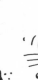

GOLD WATCH:

PAMPERING AT HEALTH SPA:

But I STILL can't forgive you for having that affair!

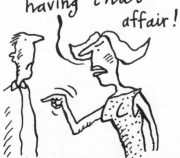

See also: BLISS (MARITAL).

**ALBATROSS** ~ Don't kill one.

**ALCOHOL** ~ See DRINKING.

**ALIBI** ~ Make sure it's a good one if you're either having an affair or planning to murder your partner who's having an affair.

# A

AGEING ~ What can I say about this? It happens to us all and it's JUST NOT FAIR!! The first real sign is when you suddenly wake up one morning to find you've become a grown-up.

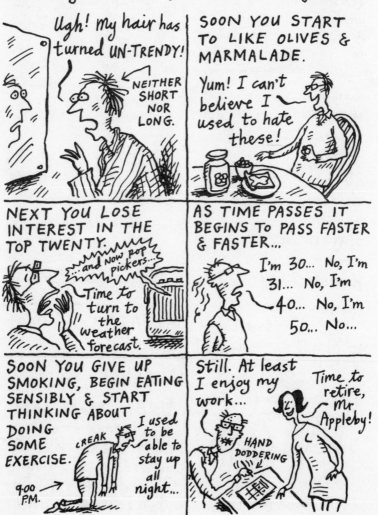

Ugh! My hair has turned UN-TRENDY!

NEITHER SHORT NOR LONG.

SOON YOU START TO LIKE OLIVES & MARMALADE.

Yum! I can't believe I used to hate these!

NEXT YOU LOSE INTEREST IN THE TOP TWENTY.

...and now Pop pickers...

Time to turn to the weather forecast.

AS TIME PASSES IT BEGINS TO PASS FASTER & FASTER...

I'm 30... No, I'm 31... No, I'm 40... No, I'm 50... No...

SOON YOU GIVE UP SMOKING, BEGIN EATING SENSIBLY & START THINKING ABOUT DOING SOME EXERCISE.

CREAK

I used to be able to stay up all night...

9.00 P.M.

Still. At least I enjoy my work...

Time to retire, Mr Appleby!

HAND DODDERING

**ALIENATION** ~ This word derives from ALIEN NATION. A race of people from a distant star system who crashed on the earth and live among us. ALIENATION describes the way they feel so far from their home planet and isolated among the strangers they will one day destroy and replace. Oh, will the rest of the invasion fleet never arrive? Will they ever see their eggs and larvae again?

See also: ABDUCTION; SEX WITH ALIENS.

AN ALIEN IN THE POST OFFICE

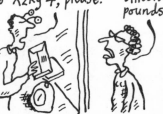

**ALLERGIES** ~ A physical response, such as sneezing, itching, dying, etc. ALLERGIES are caused by a tiny alien gun which resembles a ball-point pen.

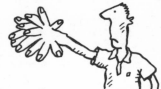

**ALL FINGERS & THUMBS** ~ Can be cured by amputation.

BEFORE:

AFTER:

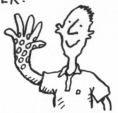

**AMNESIA** ~ Another sign that your memory has been tampered with by aliens.

# A

AGEING ~ The problem of ageing cannot be over-emphasised! It is another cause of AMNESIA.

ANAEMIA ~ Not enough blood. The answer is to drink some - if possible from a virgin.

ANGER ~ A very unpleasant and destructive emotion which should be repressed at all times. When some complete idiot annoys you, as my friend often does me, just grit your teeth, clench your fists, let your eyes bug out and your face turn bright red. Hold this for a moment. Next,

allow a low howl to escape from between your rigid jaws. By now the first tidal wave of anger should be passing.

POSITION 1 ~ Grrrr...

Allow your jaws to relax into a smile, at the same time turning the growl into light-hearted laughter.

POSITION 2 ~ He he he he... NOTE RELAXED POSTURE

Your friend will have noticed nothing, the imbecile! Other techniques for curbing anger include going home, turning to this page in the book and reading 1 2 3 4 5 6 7 8 9 10 aloud. Feel better?

22

ANTI-SOCIAL BEHAVIOUR ~ Here we see Maud distancing herself from her friends.

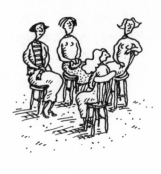

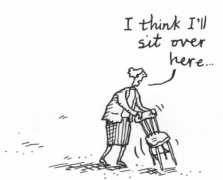

I think I'll sit over here...

This is another way of dealing with ANGER.

---

APOCALYPSE ~ The end of the world. Rather larger than most of the problems in this book, but look on the bright side. It only happens once. Unlike piles.

ARSONIST ~ Shortened form of the cry "Look at the arse on it!" (Please don't think I am being sexist. I'm not. I just report life as I find it, without comment)

# A

## ASHES ~ The result of meeting an ARSONIST. See also: DEATH.

THE ASHES OF A POOR PERSON:

THE ASHES OF A VERY RICH PERSON:

THE ASHES OF A FAMOUS PERSON — THIS IS JAMES MASON:

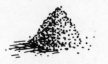

THE ASHES OF AN ORDINARY PERSON FROM NUMBER 7 UP THE ROAD:

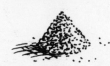

THE ASHES OF MY CAT:

ASHES OF A MOUSE ↓

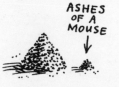

THE ASHES OF TWENTY COPIES OF THIS BOOK:

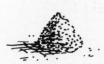

---

# WHAT TO DO WITH ASHES. Why not have them added to concrete?

Dad's in the patio.

GASP! You mean UNDER?!

No. Mixed in.

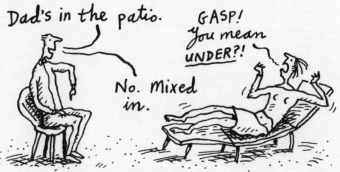

# ANTHROPOMORPHISM ~ Many people have the problem of attributing their pet cat or dog with human characteristics. I find it helpful to think of my family in animal terms. Why don't you try it?

MY WIFE IS A LIONESS.

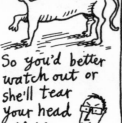

So you'd better watch out or she'll tear your head off!

OUR KIDS ARE A GOAT & THREE CHICKENS, SO THERE'S NO SHORTAGE OF MILK & EGGS IN OUR HOUSE.

Baaa!

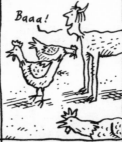

WE WANTED TO TRY FOR A COCKROACH, BUT IF WE'D HAD A FOURTH CHICKEN THAT WOULD BE TOO MANY.

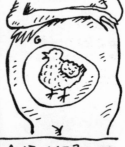

WE KEEP TWO PET HUMANS WHO PAY THEIR WAY BY AMUSING THE CHILDREN.

Peck Jim's ear!

How old is Patch in chicken years?

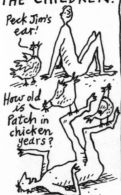

THEY'VE BEEN 'DONE', OF COURSE, AND ARE BOTH RATHER FAT.

YAWN...   Let's sleep all day!

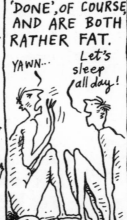

PATCH   JIM

AND ME? WELL, I'M A STICK-INSECT...

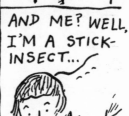

Hey! Watch where you're standing!

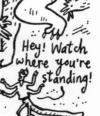

# A

## AM I GAY? ~
Probably, yes, since you've chosen to look this up. So go on, admit it to yourself and turn to COMING OUT & GAY.

## ANUS ~
A truly fascinating orifice with many exciting uses. Sadly the publishers are puritan killjoys and have censored this entry. Keep it clean and oil once a day with petroleum jelly.

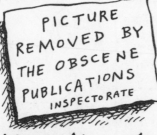

PICTURE REMOVED BY THE OBSCENE PUBLICATIONS INSPECTORATE

## ASEXUAL ~
The ideal human state to be in. We'd all get lots more done without the distraction of sex and children. Soon the human race would die out leaving the planet to the animals, plants and insects. Perfect.

Let's start inventing machines, nuclear power, cars and so on...

## AVARICE ~
Obviously we all want lots of money and possessions. I know I do. What's wrong with that? It's not a problem. I don't know how AVARICE got into this book! See also: GREED.

## AGEING ~
I make no apology for returning to this ghastly blight once again. It affects all life — particularly me. There is no cure. Just try to ignore it.

## BACK STRAIN
~ Avoid back strain by doing NO physical exercise or work whatsoever. Alternatively, if you must do something like gardening, try using these tiny garden tools...

Look - the tiny spade digs beautifully! With no risk to your back!

Space saving, too! Just pop them into your cutlery drawer along with the lawnmower, wheelbarrow and so on.

Well, must get on. I have to dig my vegetable patch over...

## BAD BREATH
~ The human body takes in pure, clean air which it processes and expels again after having added rotting food particles and odours. People inhabited by evil spirits have particularly fetid and noxious breath. Tooth-washing and gargling are useless. Beheading may work. See also: DEMONIC POSSESSION.

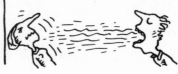

# B

BAD HAIR — Hair loyalty is something we all expect, so BAD HAIR is a very serious problem. Afterall, your hair is on display for all to see and its behaviour reflects back upon the owner. Here are some delinquent hairstyles to watch out for:

### NAUGHTY HAIR

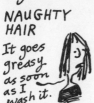

It goes greasy as soon as I wash it.

### DECEITFUL HAIR

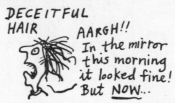

AARGH!! In the mirror this morning it looked fine! But NOW...

### CRIMINAL HAIR

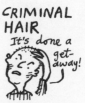

It's done a get-away!

### SCHEMING HAIR

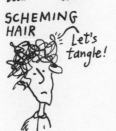

Let's tangle!

### TWO-FACED HAIR

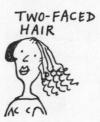

### EVIL HAIR

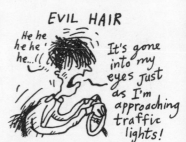

He he he he ' he...((

It's gone into my eyes just as I'm approaching traffic lights!

A professional can help you achieve good, honest... even angelic hair. Go and see your hair policeman before things get out of hand!

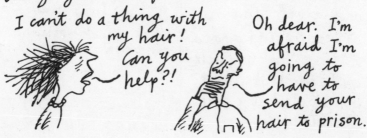

I can't do a thing with my hair! Can you help?!

Oh dear. I'm afraid I'm going to have to send your hair to prison.

# BAGGAGE

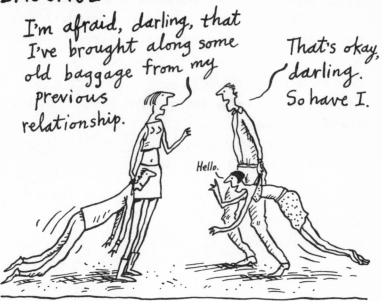

I'm afraid, darling, that I've brought along some old baggage from my previous relationship.

That's okay, darling. So have I.

Hello.

# BALDNESS ~ Men! Look forward to going bald! It's a marvellous chance to start having fun with wigs! Get a different wig for each day of the week - but don't stop there! Buy wigs for sleeping in, going out to the

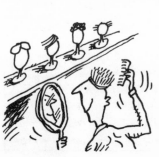

theatre, on holiday, up Everest! The sky's the limit, but don't forget that special wig to wear when flying in a jet aircraft. You'll need warm winter wigs and lighter wigs for summer. I even have a special wig for wearing in the bath which I can shampoo when I'm feeling nostalgic for the old days. Or rather, my friend has. I personally have a marvellous head of thick, black hair. So my friend's advice is: at the first sign of balding, shave off all your hair and pop down to your nearest APPLEBY'S WIG-WEAR HOUSE! Other wiggeries simply don't compare — so don't compare them! And spare a pitying thought for women. They don't go bald, poor things.

See also: BAD HAIR.

## BALLOON MODELLING

~This is a rather tragic career.
Few top fashion designers work with balloons and their impracticality for everyday wear limits their appearance in the high street. The catwalk model who specialises in balloon-wear spends most of her time sitting at home waiting for the phone to ring.

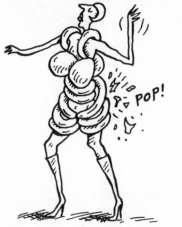

A BALLOON DRESS IS WORN TO AN EXCITING NIGHTCLUB OPENING.

## BARBER ~ See also: BAD HAIR.

## BEASTIALITY ~ A
love for cats, dogs & other beasts. Britain is a nation of beastialists. Lovers of blood sports are beastial necrophiliacs.

## BED ~ Cold and
repellent at night when one needs comfort and warmth, yet warm and nest-like in the morning when one needs to face the new day.

My bed conspires against me. I have developed plans for a bed which starts toasty warm, soft and comfy, flattening to a stiff, hardened board without covers by morning to facilitate rising.

31

# B

## BED-WETTING ~

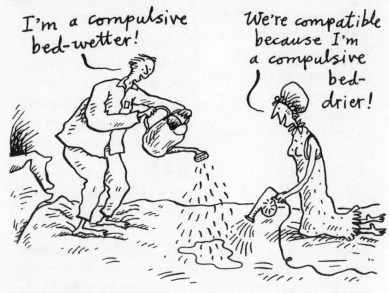

I'm a compulsive bed-wetter!

We're compatible because I'm a compulsive bed-drier!

## BEING BORING ~ You can be boring in many different ways. What you say, what you do, what you wear, what you eat, what car you drive, what tunes you whistle... the list is endless.

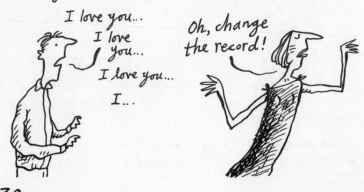

I love you...
I love you...
I love you...
I...

Oh, change the record!

Try behaving unpredictably – a difficult concept for VERY boring people. Talk about a subject you know nothing about, or order at random from a take-away menu. To help you assess your boringness levels, here's a questionnaire.

| ASPECTS OF YOUR LIFE | CRIMINALLY BORING | EXCRUCIATINGLY BORING | VERY BORING | BORING | BLAND | INTERESTING | VERY INTERESTING | INNOVATIONAL | SO EXCITING YOU COULD PRESENT A TV PROGRAMME! |
|---|---|---|---|---|---|---|---|---|---|
| HAIR | | | | | | | | | |
| TASTE IN CLOTHES | | | | | | | | | |
| TOPICS OF CONVERSATION | | | | | | | | | |
| INTERESTS | | | | | | | | | |
| SENSE OF HUMOUR | | | | | | | | | |
| FAVOURITE FILMS | | | | | | | | | |
| FAVOURITE TV | | | | | | | | | |
| JOB | | | | | | | | | |
| CAR | | | | | | | | | |
| SEXUAL SKILLS | | | | | | | | | |
| | | | | | | | | | |
| | | | | | | | | | |

# B

## BELCHING ~
WRONG!

BRROAK!!

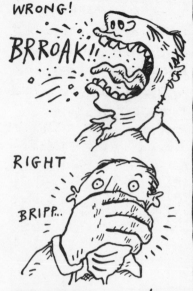

RIGHT

BRIPP...

BELCHING is nature's way of saying you're an ill-mannered slob.

## BELLY ~ Rhymes
with JELLY. There are many wobbly & bloated variations on the basic belly. A common one is the BEER BELLY. One of the rarest is the FLAT BELLY.

## BELLY BUTTON ~
This once neglected little crater comes in many forms - and many of the female ones are now visible due to the crop tops of fashion.

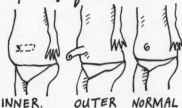

INNER.     OUTER     NORMAL

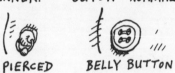

PIERCED     BELLY BUTTON

## BELOW-THE-BELT ~
An area yet to be the focus of fickle fashion. Its day will come.

STYLES TO LOOK OUT FOR

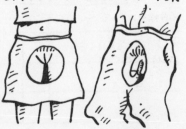

**BIKINI** ~ In the interest of fairness I have designed a male version to complement the female bikini. Such a fine item of clothing should be the property of all, not hogged by one sex (or species, for that matter).

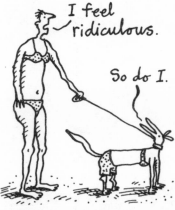

I feel ridiculous.

So do I.

**BILLS** ~ Bank managers meet once a month to ensure that the bills exceed my meagre bank balance.

See also: CASH.

**BISEXUAL** ~ A person who likes sex with both men and women. And why not. Of course, once you've successfully become a bisexual you'll find yourself looking enviously at TRISEXUALS. Then QUADSEXUALS. Or so my friend tells me.

HOW THEY MEET: HERE, FOR THE FIRST TIME, I REVEAL THE SECRET CODE PHRASE USE BY TRISEXUALS.

Have a nice day!

See also: GAY.

**BLOWING NOSE ONTO PAVEMENT** ~ This is disgusting! Don't do it! Use your shirt, underwear... ANYTHING but do this. Ugh.

**BLOND** ~ Everyone should try going blond once in their life. Before taking the plunge, simulate blondness by wearing

# B

a white pair of knickers on your head. You'll be surprised by the reactions you get!

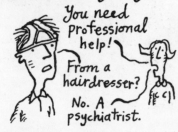

You need professional help!

From a hairdresser?

No. A psychiatrist.

**BODY** ~ See APPENDIX. (NOT the tubular sac attached to the large intestine but the APPENDIX at the back of this book).

**BODY ODOUR** ~ We all smell. It's just that some of us (myself included) smell nice and others (such as my friend) smell terrible. Wash alot and use lots of scent. Keep very still to prevent sweating.

See also: SMELLING OF CHEESE.

## BLINKERED ~

This isn't a problem at all - I LOVE it! Particularly when it's combined with

## BONDAGE ~

See: FETISHES.

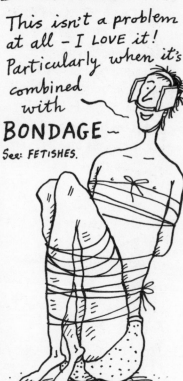

**BOIL** ~ A close-up view of a BOIL.

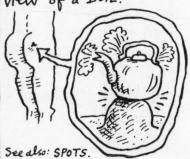

See also: SPOTS.

# BOTTOM ~

Why is my bottom called my bottom? It's in the MIDDLE of me!

Many people, often women, are very sensitive about their bottoms. So to take your mind off your own bottom difficulties (you probably need cosmetic surgery) here are some bottoms from around the universe:

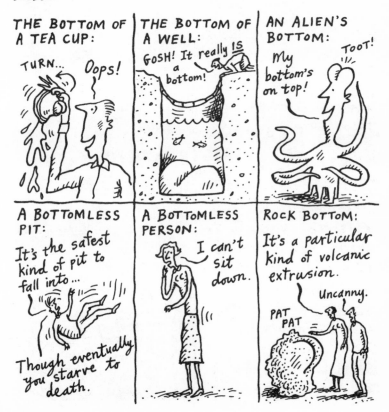

**THE BOTTOM OF A TEA CUP:**

TURN... Oops!

**THE BOTTOM OF A WELL:**

GOSH! It really IS a bottom!

**AN ALIEN'S BOTTOM:**

My bottom's on top!

TOOT!

**A BOTTOMLESS PIT:**

It's the safest kind of pit to fall into...

Though eventually you starve to death.

**A BOTTOMLESS PERSON:**

I can't sit down.

**ROCK BOTTOM:**

It's a particular kind of volcanic extrusion.

Uncanny.

PAT PAT

# B

**BOX** — A useful device for those with a very serious problem. Keep one handy to climb into in case of emergency.

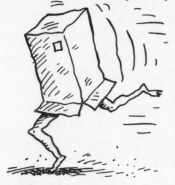

See also: PAGES 10 & 11.

**BREAST FIXATION** — Only really a problem for tranvestites, who need to fix their artificial breasts to their chests with glue. They get fixated about it. Remember to shave before sticking!
See also: FETISHES.

**BRIDLE** — Useful in BONDAGE. Don't forget the reins and saddle. Oh, and bring along some sugar cubes.
See also: FETISHES.

**BREATHING** — An offence in some families where air is in short supply.

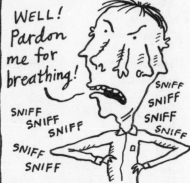

WELL! Pardon me for breathing!

SNIFF SNIFF SNIFF
SNIFF SNIFF SNIFF
SNIFF SNIFF SNIFF
SNIFF SNIFF

**BROTHER** — See FAMILY.

**BULLYING** —

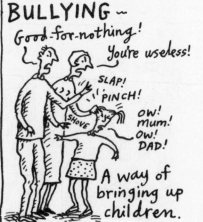

Good-for-nothing!
You're useless!
SLAP!
PINCH!
SHOVE
OW! mum!
OW! DAD!

A way of bringing up children.

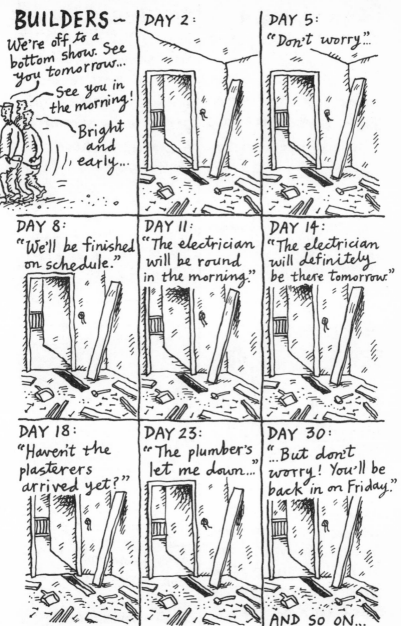

# C

**CANNIBALISM** ~ The only problem is that it is illegal. However, in today's overcrowded and permissive society I'm sure it won't be long before you're on my menu, or vice versa. And I'm sure we'd both taste delicious. Serve with green salad.

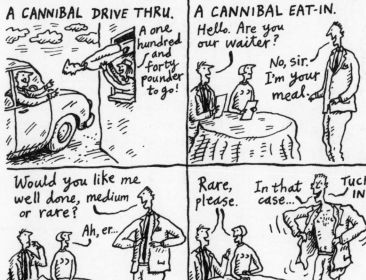

A CANNIBAL DRIVE THRU.

A one hundred and forty pounder to go!

A CANNIBAL EAT-IN.

Hello. Are you our waiter?

No, sir. I'm your meal.

Would you like me well done, medium or rare?

Ah, er...

Rare, please.

In that case...

TUCK IN!

**CAN'T** ~ There is no such word. Stop whining ~ you can do whatever you want! Even if others DON'T want you to. Just look at me!

**CAPRICIOUSNESS** ~

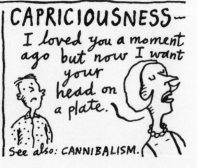

I loved you a moment ago but now I want your head on a plate.

See also: CANNIBALISM.

CARDS — Fill these in and cut them out. Keep them in your wallet or handbag and give them to your girl or boyfriends, employers, etcetera. It's always good to be open about your problems — particularly if they are not immediately visible.

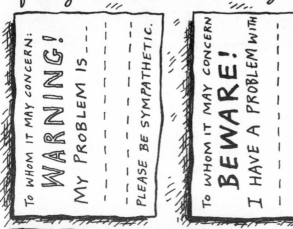

**Card 1:** TO WHOM IT MAY CONCERN: WARNING! MY PROBLEM IS ------ PLEASE BE SYMPATHETIC.

**Card 2:** TO WHOM IT MAY CONCERN BEWARE! I HAVE A PROBLEM WITH ------ PLEASE KEEP YOUR DISTANCE!

CAREER PROSPECTS — A problem for many people is: "What does my future hold?" Well, here's the answer!

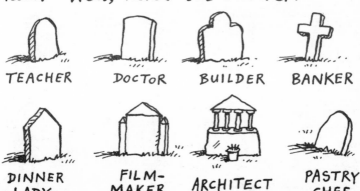

TEACHER

DOCTOR

BUILDER

BANKER

DINNER LADY

FILM-MAKER

ARCHITECT

PASTRY CHEF

C

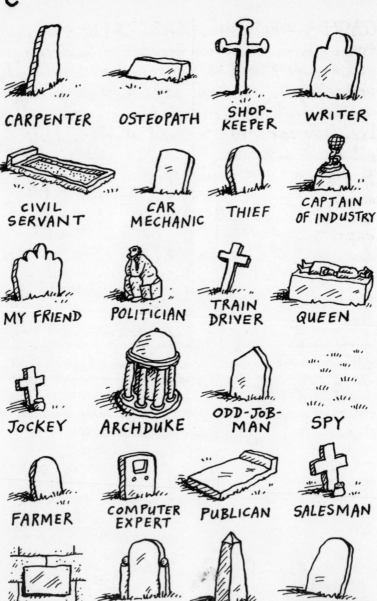

CARPENTER  OSTEOPATH  SHOP-KEEPER  WRITER

CIVIL SERVANT  CAR MECHANIC  THIEF  CAPTAIN OF INDUSTRY

MY FRIEND  POLITICIAN  TRAIN DRIVER  QUEEN

JOCKEY  ARCHDUKE  ODD-JOB-MAN  SPY

FARMER  COMPUTER EXPERT  PUBLICAN  SALESMAN

HOUSE WIFE  ACTOR  SURGEON

[FILL IN YOUR JOB]

**CASH** ~ What my friend will NOT be getting, despite his protestations, for his contributions to MY book! Friendship is all about generously giving up time (and money) for one another without expecting anything in return. This is an important lesson for him.

See also: LAWYERS!

**CASTRATION** ~ Beware of barbed-wire fences.

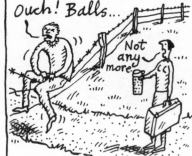

Ouch! Balls...

Not any more.

**CATALEPSY** ~ Death-like sleep in cats.

Actually, Jim IS dead!

**CATS** ~ When your cat has died you will want to buy a new one. Make sure you get a cat bred for living in a domestic home. At the kitten stage cats are cute, fluffy and playful. But BEWARE! Some cats grow into huge beasts totally unsuited to living in a small pensioner's flat — but if you have the space, they can still be loving pets.

AN AFFECTIONATE CAT:

A HUGE, SWEET-NATURED CAT:

[NOTE HAIR LICKED OFF HEAD]

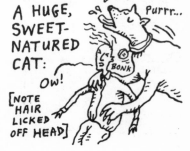

Oof! Purrrr... THUD!

Purrr... BONK Ow!

# C

## A VAST, FAT FLUFFY CAT:

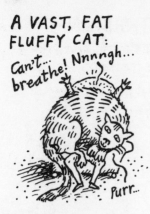

Can't... breathe! Nnnngh...

Purr...

## A COLOSSAL, CUDDLY CAT:

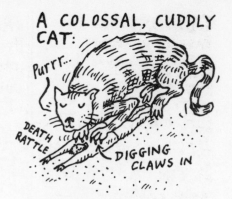

Purrr...

DEATH RATTLE

DIGGING CLAWS IN

## AN ENORMOUS, ADORABLE CAT:

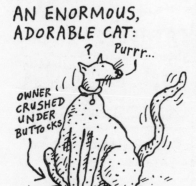

? Purrr...

OWNER CRUSHED UNDER BUTTOCKS

## A GIGANTIC, FRIENDLY CAT:

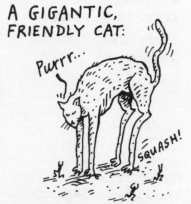

Purrr...

SQUASH!

## A STONKING GREAT FUN-LOVING CAT:

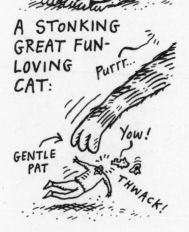

Purrr...

Yow!

GENTLE PAT

THWACK!

## A GARGANTUAN HAPPY OLD CAT STUCK UP A TREE:

That's it - Jump down into my arms, Woosums... AARGH!!

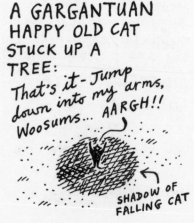

SHADOW OF FALLING CAT

**CELIBACY** ~ See CASTRATION; ASEXUAL.

**CELLULITE** ~ See COSMETIC SURGERY.

**CHILDREN** ~ When I was a child myself other children existed only to shun, ridicule and bully me. Now, in later life they have been given powerful positions in the government, police force and banking profession where they continue to ridicule, bully and shun me. I suspect my own offspring to be aliens operating in another time continuum, returning to our own dimension to vomit just as I drop into deep sleep.
It is traditional, at the end of the summer holidays, for parents to dance the celebratory 'Back to school' Gay Gordon around a bonfire on which they burn a wicker child.

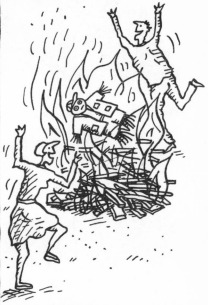

**CHRISTMAS** ~ A punishment devised for people who have children.

**CLOSET** ~ See: COMING OUT.
See also your local furniture store and catalogue. Here's a

# C

sexy self-assembly closet.

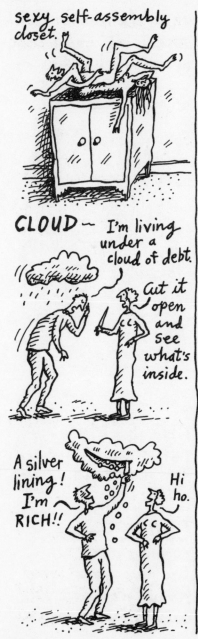

## CLOUD ~
I'm living under a cloud of debt.

Cut it open and see what's inside.

A silver lining! I'm RICH!!

Hi ho.

## COLD FEET ~

Darling, I'm afraid I've got cold feet...

Oh, thank God! So have I! Let's call the wedding off!

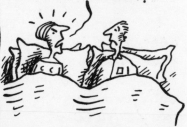

No. I meant my FEET are cold!!

Bad circulation to the feet can cause temporary discomfort, but bad circulation to the brain causes permanent impairment of the faculties.

**COMING OUT** ~ There are a number of
different ways to come out. Let's take
a closer look...

**COMING OUT OF
THE CLOSET:**

Did you find what
you were looking
for?   I found myself!

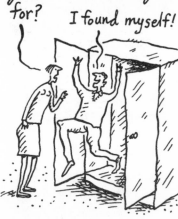

**COMING OUT OF
A SHOP:**

I've bought a
lovely frock!

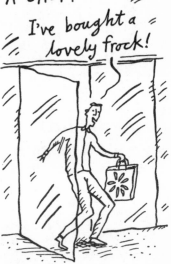

**COMING OUT OF
FIONA:**

UGH! Yuk!!

At least you
won't get
pregnant!

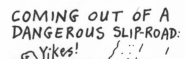

**COMING OUT OF A
DANGEROUS SLIP-ROAD:**

Yikes!

SLAM!  BAM!  CRUNCH!

THUD

Serves
him right
for
coming out!

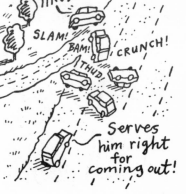

# COMPLEX—

I've got a terrible complexion!

You've just got a complex.

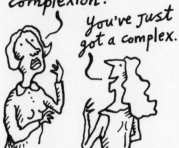

# COMPLEXION—

Oops! No, you're right. You haven't got a complex. You HAVE got a terrible complexion!

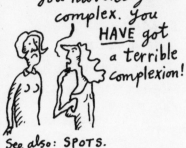

See also: SPOTS.

# COMPULSIONS —

MR A HAS A COMPULSION TO CALL HIMSELF 'DIANA'.

Hi!

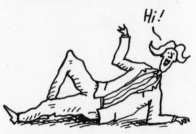

MR B HAS A COMPULSION TO CALL OTHER PEOPLE 'DIANA'.

Hello, Diana.

How kind. In fact my real name is Bob.

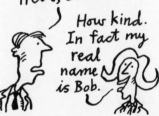

MR C FEELS COMPELLED TO CALL ANYONE NAMED DIANA 'BOB'.

I just can't help myself, Bob!

No harm done.

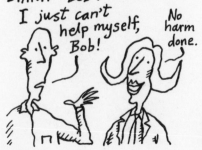

IF MR A, B & C MEET, HOW MANY 'DIANAS' WILL THERE BE AND HOW MANY 'BOBS'?

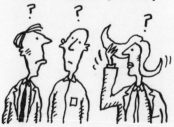

C

**COMPUTER GAMES-**
This is a new-fangled problem so I'm not an expert, but basically you need the latest super-fast video card, processor, ram, hard drive and internet connection or you'll have terrible problems with your teenager.

Aw Dad! Our computer's CRAP! Our modem's RUBBISH! I hate you!!

**CONDOM** - give your teenager some of these in an attempt to distract him from computer games.

**CONTRACEPTION ~**
Castration is probably the most effective form of contraception,

although same-sex sex has a good success rate too. After that I recommend celibacy or having children. Both are pretty effective at preventing pregnancy.

Mum! Dad! What are you doing? Nothing. Now!

See also: CHILDREN.

**COSMETIC SURGERY~**
We all have room for improvement, so why not book into Doctor Bob's Cosmetic Carvery. (Incidentally, 'Doctor' is Mr Bob's first name, NOT a qualification). Doctor Bob is delighted to work

49

# C

on cats, dogs and other pets as well as humans, so bring them along. And take advantage of Bob's 'TWO FOR THE PRICE OF JUST YOU!' special deal.

CAT NOSE JOB:

BEFORE          AFTER

Doctor Bob can make your pet bigger, smaller, thinner, fatter, balder or hairier – just as he can for you, too.

BEFORE          AFTER

To give you confidence, let me point out that Doctor Bob has also operated on his own face perfectly successfully.

**COWS** ~ Being large creatures, cows have even bigger personal problems than we do. I put that thought into the book to make you feel better about yourself. It always works for me.

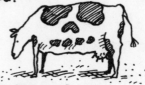

DEPRESSED COW

**COWARDICE** ~ A yellow streak running down the spine. Not dangerous. In fact, quite the opposite. Many cowards live long and happy lives.

**CRABS** ~ Tiny creatures who live under rocks in pools on our groin beaches. See also: GROIN LOBSTER.

# CRAZES ~
## A CRAZE BEGINNING & ENDING

**IN THE MORNING:**

I'm OBSESSED with GLUING FELT!

**AT LUNCHTIME:**

Now I'm bored with it.

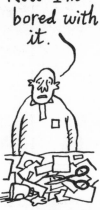

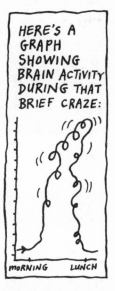

HERE'S A GRAPH SHOWING BRAIN ACTIVITY DURING THAT BRIEF CRAZE:

MORNING    LUNCH

HERE'S AN UNUSUAL CRAZE:

We wear our hair upside down!

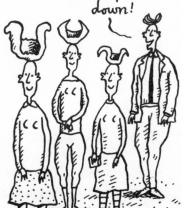

SOME CRAZES ARE CRAZY! MRS SPOT HAS STARTED A CRAZE FOR SPONGING DOWN STAN:

It hasn't really caught on yet.

Except with you, Agnes.

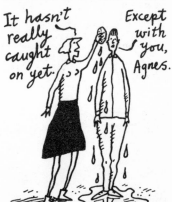

51

# CREDIT CARDS ~

CREDIT CARDS are marvellous! They allow you to spend 'invisible' money which they draw from bank accounts in a parallel universe. Unfortunately the inhabitants of the other universe ALSO have credit cards which take money from YOUR bank account. Try to stay ahead of the people from the other world by spending as fast as you can!

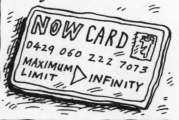

# CROSS-DRESSING ~

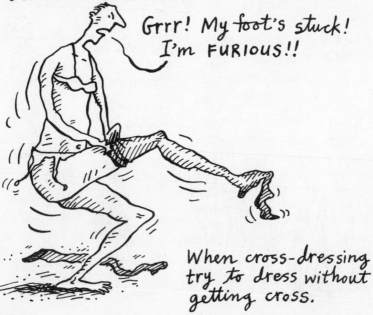

Grrr! My foot's stuck! I'm FURIOUS!!

When cross-dressing try to dress without getting cross.

CULTS ~ Beware of cults. Many of them are run by charlatans and frauds who are only interested in taking your money! To help you avoid a costly mistake, my friend and I have started our own END OF THE WORLD cults which you can join with impunity (and a small fee for administration). Choose from one of the three below.

① THE CHURCH OF TAME FLYING ANTS.

Tame your ant well, my son.

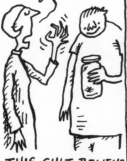

THIS CULT BELIEVE THAT WHEN THE WORLD ENDS ANTS WILL GROW HUGE AND ONLY THOSE PEOPLE WITH A TAME ANT WILL BE CARRIED TO SAFETY.

② THE CHILDREN OF DONUTS, POP AND CRISPS.

Eat, eat and eat again, brothers!

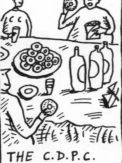

THE C.D.P.C. BELIEVE THAT FLYING-SAUCER PEOPLE ARE COMING TO CHOOSE THE PLUMPEST OF US FOR THE HONOUR OF BEING ALIEN FOOD.

③ THE TEMPLE OF DECEIT.

The WORLD is about to END!

REALLY?!

No!

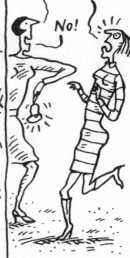

SEND YOUR MONEY %: THE PUBLISHERS.

# D

**DADDY** ~ see FAMILY.

**DADDY (SUGAR)** ~ Keep away from water or he will dissolve to nothing.

**DANDRUFF** ~ Flakes of skin falling off your head. This is a miracle, like the loaves and fishes. Our scalps are finite but dandruff is infinite. It just keeps on coming.

**DANGEROUS CUSTOMS** ~ Stubble burning.

We set light to each other's beard stubble!

YIPPEE!

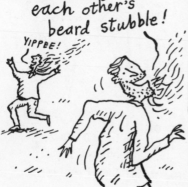

**DARK SIDE** ~ We all have a dark side. Go on, admit it!

Your side is only dark because you don't WASH properly!

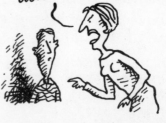

I can't see to read!

You're sitting on my DARK SIDE!

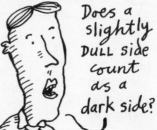

Does a slightly DULL side count as a dark side?

54

**DEATH** ~ We're all afraid of death, me included. A helpful tip is not to think about it. Taking that approach one step further, many people find they can pretend that it's never going to happen. Until...

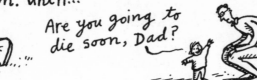

Are you going to die soon, Dad?

**SOME DAYS I'M PREPARED FOR IT.**

Right! I've had a shower, washed the dishes and paid the bills!

**OTHER DAYS I'M NOT.**

Haven't finished this book yet!

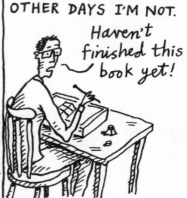

**I GUESS MY TIME WILL COME WHETHER I'M READY OR NOT.**

Tsk! He didn't finish his life's work!

Lazy so and so!

MY AGENT

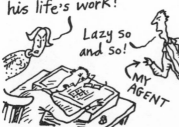

**SO MY ADVICE IS: BE PREPARED - JUST IN CASE.**

Ugh! Dad didn't wash behind his ears!

Or brush his teeth!

Look! Here's his porn collection!

# D

# HOW TO TELL IF DEATH
# HAS OCCURRED:

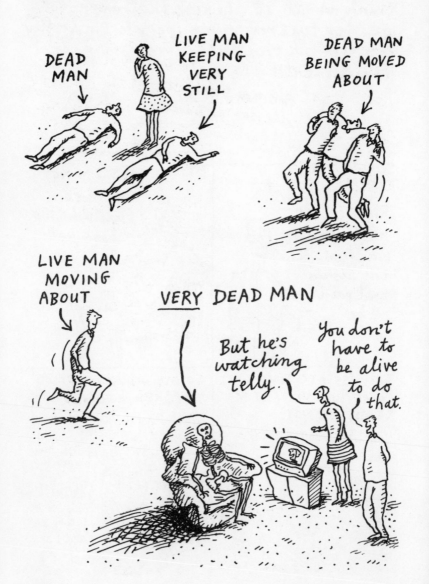

**DECEIT** ~ Including **DESPAIR & DIVORCE**
See also: AFFAIR.

**DELUDING YOURSELF** ~ The fact that you are looking this up is a good sign. At worst you're still deluding yourself that you're no longer deluding yourself. At best you're on the road to recovery. Of course, deluding myself was never my problem. See also: IN DENIAL.

# DELUSIONS ~

A MAN WHO THINKS HE'S A HIPPO

A HIPPO WHO THINKS HE'S A MAN

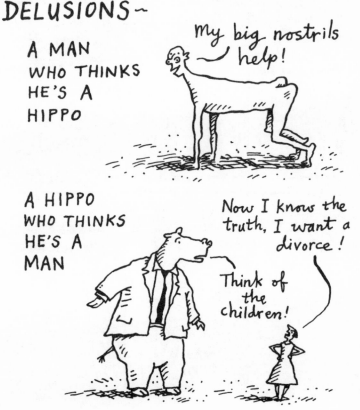

# D

## DEMONIC POSSESSION ~ A cautionary tale!

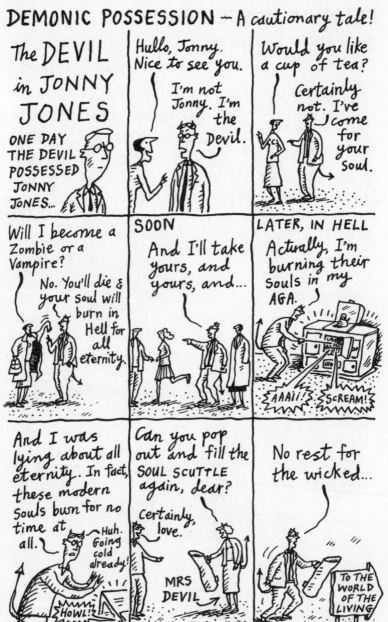

# DEMONIC POSSESSIONS ~

A HOLIDAY HOME POSSESSED BY THE DEVIL:

*I bought it for when I need a break.*

SOME OF THE DEVIL'S OTHER POSSESSIONS:

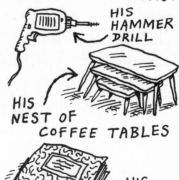

HIS HAMMER DRILL

HIS NEST OF COFFEE TABLES

HIS EXORCISE BOOK

---

DIET ~ You'll lose weight faster than you ever thought possible if you buy STEVEN APPLEBY'S range of IMAGINARY FOOD!

**BREAKFAST**

TOAST    CEREAL    BOILED EGG

**PACKED LUNCH**

SANDWICHES, CRISPS, CHOC BAR & FRUIT

**AFTERNOON TEA**

CREAM CAKES    CAKE    SCONES

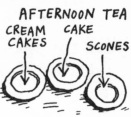

**DINNER**

NUGGETS, CHIPS & PEAS    PUD

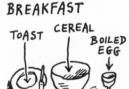

**EVEN CAT FOOD IS AVAILABLE!**

DRIED SHAPES

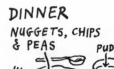

**A TYPICAL BATTLE**

*I'm full!*

*Eat your peas!*

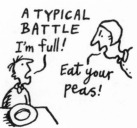

# D

## DISTINGUISHING MARKS – We

all worry about becoming an unidentified corpse and denying our loved ones the satisfaction of a funeral. Find peace of mind with a permanent distinguishing mark.

WHY NOT INVEST IN A TATTOO LIKENESS OF YOURSELF!

OR HOW ABOUT A MAP TATTOO OF THE AREA WHERE YOU LIVE?

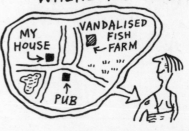

MY HOUSE

VANDALISED FISH FARM

PUB

ENHANCES YOUR APPEARANCE IN LIFE AND IDENTIFIES YOU IN THE EVENT OF DECAPITATION.

THIS LADY HAS HAD EVERY PART OF HER BODY NUMBERED AND TAGGED TO ALLOW FOR THE MOST AWFUL EVENTUALITY.

PERHAPS AN EXTRA BELLY BUTTON WILL DO THE TRICK.

Not many people have an extra 6!

* GLUE GUARANTEED FOR **70** YEARS! *

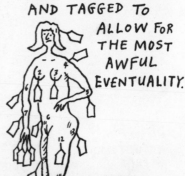

PHONE FOR A BROCHURE.

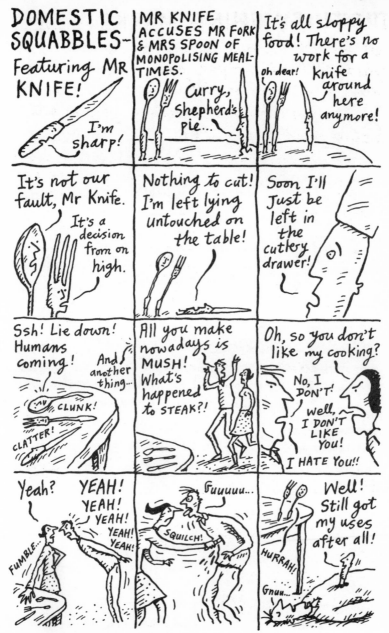

# D

## DON'T CRY WOLF!

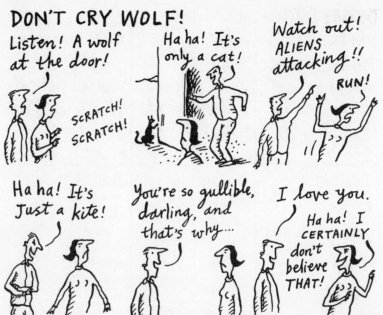

Listen! A wolf at the door!

SCRATCH! SCRATCH!

Ha ha! It's only a cat!

Watch out! ALIENS attacking!!

RUN!

Ha ha! It's just a kite!

You're so gullible, darling, and that's why...

I love you.

Ha ha! I CERTAINLY don't believe THAT!

---

**DREAMS** ~ When the voices in my head gather to perform plays. Day-dreaming should be encouraged. Shakespeare probably dreamt of being a playwright. Picasso of being an artist. Dream as often as possible. Without our dreams we would just be animals.

**DREAMING WHILE ASLEEP** ~ This is pointless and unproductive. You can never remember them so what possible use can they be? Best ignored.

I dreamt of being a... Oh, I forget....

See also: NIGHTMARES.

**DROOLING** ~ A particularly sordid habit, especially on trains and in other public places. Men also drool over dirty magazines (which is why the pages stick together) and cars (ruining the paintwork and upholsetry). Women drool over chocolate and men wearing shining armour.

The APPLEBY SLEEP-SILENT can prevent dribbling and snoring in trains.

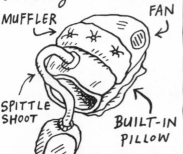

MUFFLER
FAN
SPITTLE SHOOT
BUILT-IN PILLOW

Dangerous to use, but worth it to prevent the awful embarrassment of waking up to find the whole carriage looking at you.

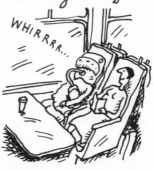

WHIRRR...

THE FAN PROMOTES AIR CIRCULATION AND PREVENTS SUFFOCATION (USUALLY). Remember to squeeze out the sponges after use.
See also: SNORING.

**DUAL PERSONALITY-**

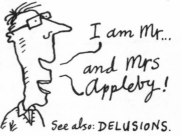

I am Mr... and Mrs Appleby!

See also: DELUSIONS.

# D

**DULLNESS** — A dull new theory suggests that dull people think in black & white while interesting, fun people think in colour. Really wacky and zany folk think in wide-screen 3-D, but let's not hop, skip and jump before we can walk. Trying to think in sepia will do for a start.

SOME DULL & BORING MEN:

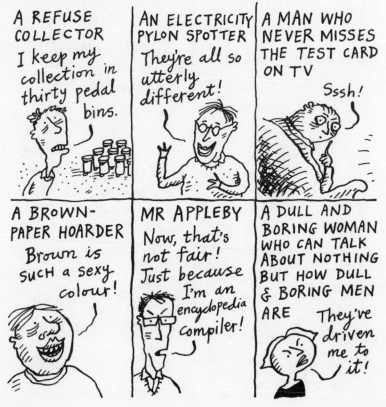

A REFUSE COLLECTOR
I keep my collection in thirty pedal bins.

AN ELECTRICITY PYLON SPOTTER
They're all so utterly different!

A MAN WHO NEVER MISSES THE TEST CARD ON TV
Sssh!

A BROWN-PAPER HOARDER
Brown is such a sexy colour!

MR APPLEBY
Now, that's not fair! Just because I'm an encyclopedia compiler!

A DULL AND BORING WOMAN WHO CAN TALK ABOUT NOTHING BUT HOW DULL & BORING MEN ARE
They've driven me to it!

# E

**EAR WAX** ~ Used to hold an ear wig in place.

**EAVESDROPPING** ~ Eve's dropping her knickers at the SLIGHTEST provocation, Aunt Bagwood. I overheard Simone say so!

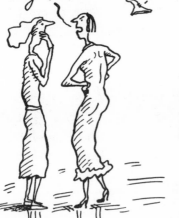

**ECCENTRICITY** ~ Being yourself, not someone else. Or rather, not what someone else thinks you should be.

**ECZEMA** ~ A skin complaint curable using Chinese herbs.

**EGOTISM** ~ Me!

**EJACULATE** ~ The opposite in conception of immaculate conception.

**EMBARRASSMENT** ~

COLD SWEAT

RED CHEEKS

GROUND OPENING

Condition caused by having to say 'ejaculate' in mixed company.

**EMOTIONAL OUT-BURST** ~

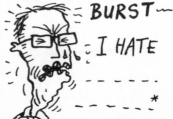

I HATE _ _ _ _ _ _ _ _ _ *

*YOU CHOOSE.

65

# E

**ENORMOUS ~**
See: PENIS.

**ENVY ~** See: PENIS.

**EPIDEMIC ~**

There's an epidemic
of PENIS
REFERENCES
around here!

See also: PENIS.

**EPILOGUE ~** There
is NO epilogue in
this book. Except
right here.

**ERECTION ~**
See: PENIS.

**ESCAPE ~** There
IS no escape.

THE TUNNEL OF
LIFE LEADS
ONLY TO
ANOTHER TUNNEL.

**ETIQUETTE ~** A mine-field booby-trapped
with bowls of soup for you to put your
feet into. My advice is to copy what
everyone else does, until you notice
that no one is doing anything —
because they are ALL following my
advice. Now you can safely eat without worrying. Go on! Lick your knife!
Because ETIQUETTE is too large a
subject to cover in detail here, I'll
confine myself to one crucial subject:
SOCIAL KISSING. Follow these directions
and the first impression you make
will be a good one.

# THE LANGUAGE of SOCIAL KISSING

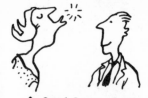

A SINGLE AIR KISS ~ 'I can't remember, who you are.'

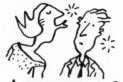

A DOUBLE AIR KISS ~ 'My lipstick is more important than you.'

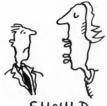

SHOULD YOU KISS THIS LADY ONCE, TWICE OR THREE TIMES?

How do you do?

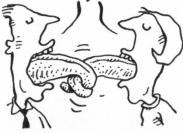

THE 'HANDSHAKE' ~ Traditional yet informal.

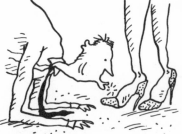

THE SHOE SHINE ~ Deferential & polite.

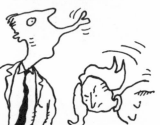

THE DUCK ~ 'I never liked you.'

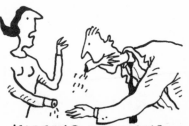

KISSING THE HAND ~ 'Watch out. I'm a weirdo!'

# E

**EVIL** — See: EXAMS.

**EXAMS** — See: EVIL.

**EXCUSES** — "I'm doing my best in this book," I said to my friend. "I can't try any harder!" "There's no such word as 'can't'," he raged. "And anyway, I'll do it if you can't, then <u>I'll</u> get all the money." I frowned. He was right. I COULD try harder. No more excuses. And he's certainly not getting a penny! Read on...
See also: CAN'T.

**EXERCISE** — We all hate exercise. I'm hopeless at making time to go to the gym so I devised these exercises to do while dozing in a chair or lying in bed fast asleep.

POSITION ONE:
DEEP BREATHING

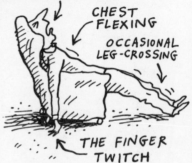

CHEST FLEXING

OCCASIONAL LEG-CROSSING

THE FINGER TWITCH

POSITION TWO:

MORE DEEP BREATHING

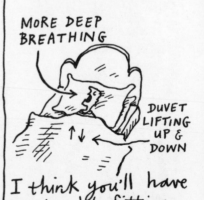

DUVET LIFTING UP & DOWN

I think you'll have no trouble fitting these exercises in.

**EXHIBITIONISM** — What I do for a living. All my thoughts and feelings are in this book thinly disguised as other people's problems. Or my friends'.

**EXOSKELETON** —

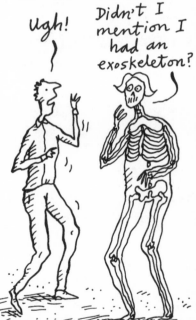

Ugh!

Didn't I mention I had an exoskeleton?

BRIAN MEETS HIS EMAIL PAL FOR THE FIRST TIME.

**EXOTIC** — Some people LIKE an exoskeleton, of course. They find it exotic.

**EXPOSÉ** — A newspaper article revealing what it is like to have an affair with someone with an exoskeleton.

**EXTINCT** — Dead and gone. It happens to all sorts of sweets (for example, Marathon), comics, television programmes, businesses, bus routes, hospitals, shops, and of course animals... the list is endless. Why on earth it hasn't happened to human beings I do not know. There's no justice.

# F

## FAILURE ~
Stop rushing about trying to imitate the successes of others. Rather than failing at things, why not be successful at doing nothing instead.

## FAILURE TO RECOGNISE AN OLD FRIEND ~

I'll take my glasses off...

I'll put my glasses on...

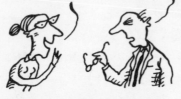

## FAIR-WEATHER FRIEND ~
Someone who won't lend you their umbrella.

Looks like hail...

Goodbye.

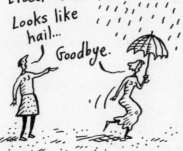

## FALSIES ~
In the future falsies will be engineered to function just like the real thing. No need to make excuses when it's time to slip out of your top or bottom.

Wow!

Wow!

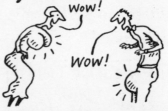

## FAIRY GODMOTHER ~

Would you like me to make your falsies real?

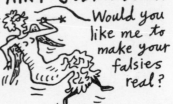

## FAIT ACCOMPLI ~

I'm moving in with my girlfriend, Dad.

I've already moved in with her, Darren.

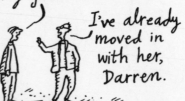

## FAME ~
A lack of fame is a problem.

**FAMILY** — Your family consists of people who are related to you. I'm sorry, but there it is. There's no getting away from it - apart from by leaving home, which many people do each year. My suggestion is that these fugitives should form their own UN-RELATED families.

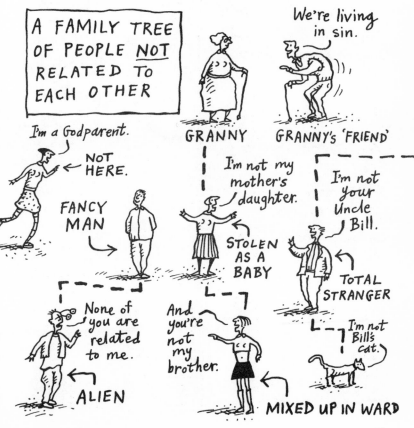

A FAMILY TREE OF PEOPLE **NOT** RELATED TO EACH OTHER

We're living in sin.

I'm a Godparent. ← NOT HERE.

GRANNY

GRANNY'S 'FRIEND'

FANCY MAN

I'm not my mother's daughter.

STOLEN AS A BABY

I'm not your Uncle Bill.

TOTAL STRANGER

None of you are related to me.

ALIEN

And you're not my brother.

I'm not Bill's cat.

MIXED UP IN WARD

71

# F

## FAMILY LIFE ~ An ordinary morning in an ordinary home.

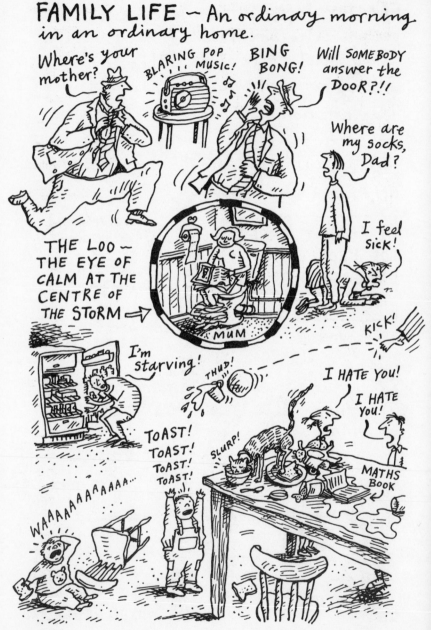

The family even put pressure on from beyond the grave. Here we see the GHOSTS of FAMILY MEMBERS PAST trying to make Myrtle feel the weight of family tradition and repent her wanton ways!

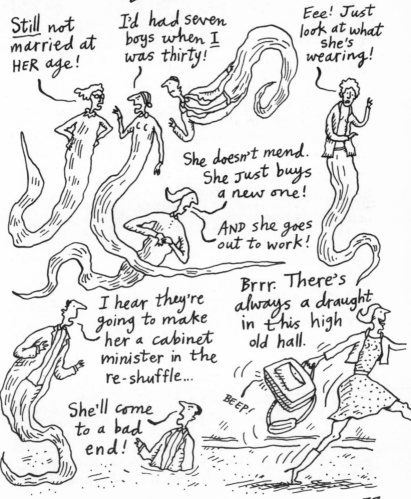

73

# F

## FANCYING SOMEONE WHO DOESN'T FANCY YOU ~

He's gorgeous!

She's Gorgonish!

See also: DELUSIONS; IN DENIAL.

## FANTASY ~

Few relationships are big enough for more than one fantasy. Take turns. It is the death of love when fantasies collide.

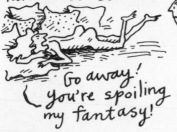

Go away! You're spoiling my fantasy!

## FARTING ~

Can be seen as positive or negative depending on the age and sex of your social group.

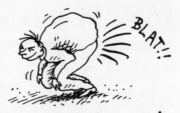

BLAT!!

Among boys and men in general farting is considered hilarious and will make you popular and well liked. The louder the better! Teenage girls and women, however, regard it as uncouth. But then, what do they know?

Oh God! I'm sorry! Pardon me...

TOOT!

## FASTING ~

Purify your system with a fast. Forty days is traditional. Alternatively, try a fast fast lasting only a few minutes, then you can gorge again at lunchtime.

# FASTENER

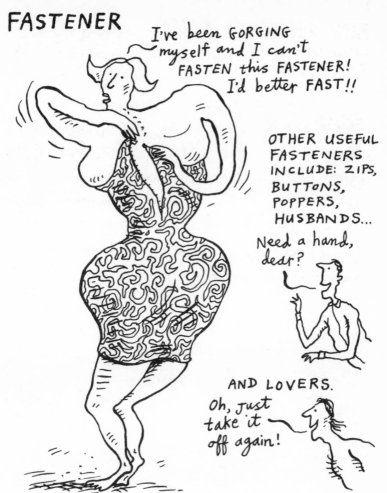

I've been GORGING myself and I can't FASTEN this FASTENER! I'd better FAST!!

OTHER USEFUL FASTENERS INCLUDE: ZIPS, BUTTONS, POPPERS, HUSBANDS...

Need a hand, dear?

AND LOVERS. Oh, just take it off again!

**FATAL** ~ Too much fasting and gorging.

**FEELING BLUE** ~ A hot bath should clean you up and raise your spirits.

**FEELING A FRIEND** ~ A mistake. Friends make complicated lovers.

**FEELING A FRIEND'S WIFE** ~ A bigger and more complicated mistake.

# F

FETISHISM — A fetish is an object or part of the anatomy which arouses libido. It could be a lady's ankle, an item of clothing, going round stately homes — even this book itself! Feel the silky-smooth vinyl cover caress your hands as you read. Smell the musky plastic odour. Mmm... Loosen your clothing. Your hands become sweaty as desire courses through your body. The book slips out of your trembling fingers and falls between your waiting thighs. Perhaps a part of the book offends you? Pinch each page as you turn it, folding the book cruelly back. Bad book. Bad Mr Appleby. Spank the book! Spank Mr Appleby! Confine the book between two large, leather volumes. Squeeze the book tight... Uh. Ah. There we are. An example. Rather far-fetched. Of a fetish. Let's move along and look at some other instances...

Good book?

Ooh, yes!

F

# BONDAGE ~ A classic fetish, much practised. Here are some ideas the beginner can try at home:

**ESPALIER TRAINING FOR MS. BROWN**

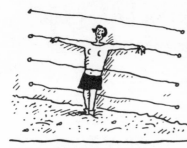

**RYAN LAYS HIS OWN CARPETS**

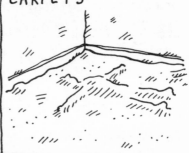

**MRS BOBBS IS A SIGN ON HER OWN BEDROOM DOOR**

KEEP OUT!

**HARRY LIKES TO DRY HIS CLOTHES WHILE HE'S WEARING THEM**

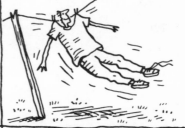

**A MAN TIED UP LIKE A PARCEL**

I'm a POSTMAN!

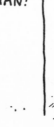

**A CASE OF HUMAN BONDAGE**

I love you and I'm NEVER going to let you go!

SQUEEZE!

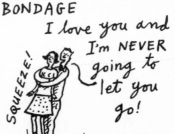

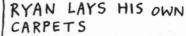

77

# F

**MORE FETISHES:**

**DENDRAPHILIAC ~**
Lover of trees.

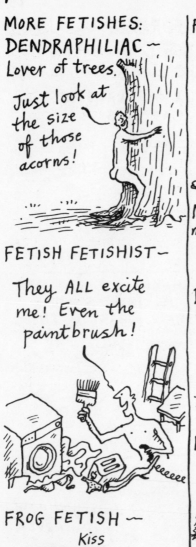

Just look at the size of those acorns!

**FETISH FETISHIST ~**

They ALL excite me! Even the paintbrush!

**FROG FETISH ~**

Kiss me!

Hop it, weirdo!

**FOOT FETISH ~**

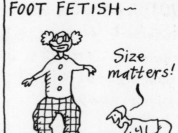

Size matters!

**MATCH FETISHIST meets CAKE FETISHIST ~**

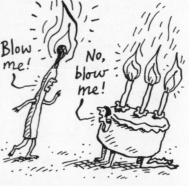

Blow me!

No, blow me!

**NECROPHILIA ~**
But I'm a ghost! It'll pass right through me!

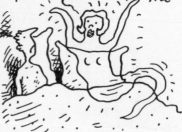

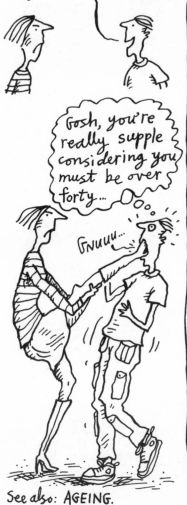

## FOOT-IN-MOUTH DISEASE ~

You look really young considering you're very old.

*Gosh, you're really supple considering you must be over forty...*

*GNUUU...*

See also: AGEING.

**FORTY** ~ You spend all your time trying to not look forty. You re-assess your life & find it wanting.

**FOSSIL** ~ What you become when you're forty.

**FREUDIAN SLIPS** ~ Undergarments worn by Sigmund Freud.

**FRIEND** ~ Person forced to help compile encyclopedia by ruthless cartoonist – or else I'll pass the information concerning the triple axe murders to the police. As well as blackmail, friends can be bought. An ideal gift for that person who's got everything. Except a friend. Another ideal present is this book.
See also: MOLE.

# F

**FRIGID** ~ Like a fridge. Look on the bright side. You can keep milk cool, chill white wine and help jelly to set. But take a good book and a hot-water bottle to bed with you rather than a sexual partner.
See also: ASEXUAL.

**FUCK UP** ~
See: FAMILY.

**FUDDY DUDDY** ~
What your children (and anyone under thirty) thinks you are when you reach forty. Surprise them! Release a hit single or two – but beware. If you fail to reach the Top 20 you'll be a 'sad' has-been.

**FUTURE** ~ There is no future.

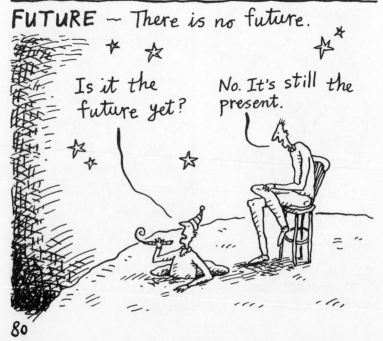

Is it the future yet?

No. It's still the present.

**GAY** — Being light-hearted. Well, I can't really see a problem with this, so if being gay makes you light-hearted then get on with it. There would be nothing worse than becoming old without having been light-hearted. What a waste.

See also: COMING OUT.

**GENDER** — What sex you are. If you are unsure about this, lift your skirt or drop your pants and take a look. Still confused? Consult these anatomical drawings or ask a friend to give you their honest opinion.

MALE & FEMALE. USUALLY

**GETTING SACKED** — Getting sacked frequently looks bad on your CV, so it is probably better not to get a job at all. You'll soon find that your fear of getting sacked disappears.

See also: FAILURE.

**GETTING UP** — A common problem. Just stay in bed until the next morning. This means that instead of getting up late on Monday, you are up bright and early on Tuesday.

# G

GENITAL ABNORMALITIES ~ No two people have identical genitals, so don't be alarmed if yours are bigger, smaller, fatter, thinner, noisier or in the wrong place compared to your colleagues' at work or mates' in the pub. Simply advertise in a specialist magazine or cut out the appropriate badge on pages 111 & 112.

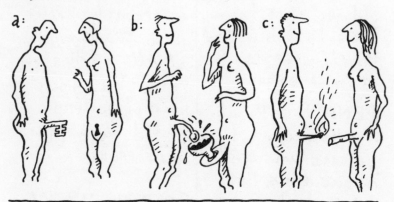

GIFTED CHILDREN ~ We've all got these!

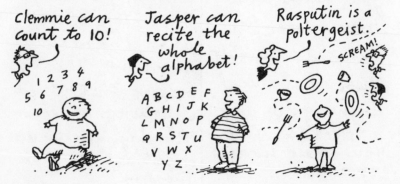

Clemmie can count to 10!

Jasper can recite the whole alphabet!

Rasputin is a poltergeist.

# GIFTED GENITALS — It's hard not to be envious when you see something like RALPH'S TALKING PENIS:

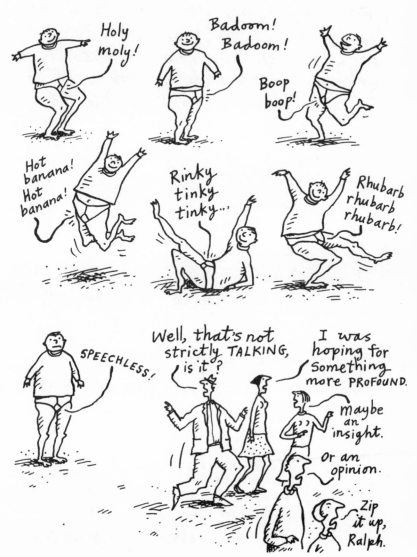

# G

## GOSSIP ~

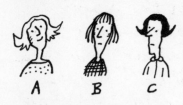

A    B    C

Appleby's General
Theory of Gossip
goes as follows:

$$a + b + c = \begin{cases} \text{MAKE} \\ \text{GENERAL} \\ \text{POLITE} \\ \text{SMALL-TALK} \end{cases}$$

$$a + b - c = \begin{cases} \text{TALK} \\ \text{ABOUT c.} \end{cases}$$

↑

FOR EXAMPLE, C
GOES TO THE LOO.

A variation on the
first equation can
be extrapolated thus:

$$a + b + c = \begin{cases} \text{TALK ABOUT} \\ \text{EVERYONE} \\ \text{WE KNOW} \\ \text{WHO ISN'T} \\ \text{HERE plus} \\ \text{SOME WE} \\ \text{DON'T} \\ \text{KNOW.} \end{cases}$$

Using the General
Theory as a starting
point, one can calculate
the likelihood of there
being BLACK HOLES of
silence, where the
density of Gossip is
so great that no
sound can escape.
This can also cause
BENDING of TIME itself!

Good God!
I completely
forgot to
pick TITUS
up from
nursery!!

GREED ~ I have a
desire to possess
YOUR money, which
is why I wrote this
book. If you are
idly browsing these
pages in a bookshop
STOP NOW! and take
the book STRAIGHT
to your nearest
checkout! Thank you...

**GRIZZLE** ~ What small children and men do when they're over-tired.

**GRUMPY** ~ A sign that you are taking things out on the people round about you instead of dealing with what is really bothering you.

---

**GUILT** ~ The emotion which holds couples and society together. Try to relieve your guilty feelings by tackling their cause. Return all that money you embezzled or talk to the person you hurt.

I feel *so* guilty that we're splitting up!

Oh, don't feel guilty about that. These things happen...

Oh thank you...

No! Feel GUILTY for WASTING the best years of MY LIFE! MY YOUTH! MY LOOKS! YOU SLIMY BASTARD!!

# H

**HAIR** ~ The little-known truth is that we are born already stuffed full of all the hair we will ever have.

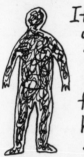

It fills us up and 'grows' slowly out from tiny holes in our skin right throughout our lives. When it runs out we go bald. We also become lighter and shrink slightly

**HALITOSIS** — See BAD BREATH.

**HATE** ~ This is a very negative and destructive emotion. You must try to bury the hatchet.

**HATCHET** ~ Let's bury the hatchet!

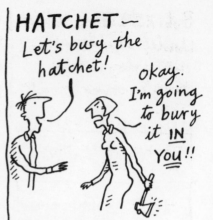

Okay. I'm going to bury it _IN_ _YOU_!!

**HAVING AN UNFORTUNATE NAME** ~ Some unlucky people had parents with a sense of humour who called them Byron, Hortense, Effigenia or Bob. But don't lose heart — it's easy to change names! Just fill in the card, photocopy it and send it to everyone you know and Bob's your Uncle... And if

Bob **REALLY** **IS** your Uncle, then why not copy some blank cards for him, too.

✂---

TO WHOM IT MAY INTEREST, I

_ _ _ _ _ _ _ _ _ _

hereby announce that from this day hence I wish to be known as

_ _ _ _ _ _ _ _ _

_ _ _ _ _ _ _ _ _

_ _ _ _ _ _ _ _

SEX: ☐ MALE ☐ FEMALE

I will pretend not to hear you if you use my old name.

**HEAD LOUSE** – The ruling louse in a tribe of lice. One particular louse is elected head and then must perform an heroic feat of courage. The Head Louse rules until washed away by organophosphate-based shampoo.

**HEART** – Fragile and easily broken. People have heart attacks, meaning they are broken-hearted.

**HEIGHT** – We are either too high, like my friend, or too low, like me. There is no happy medium.

**HERO** – Heroin for men.

**HEROIN** ~ Don't glamorise this drug! You need the best specialist treatment. Book into the entire top floor of an Hotel, hire a limo to the gig and get someone to help carry you onstage. Kick the habit when your career flags.

**HIBERNATION** ~

He's not dead, Mrs C. Just hibernating.

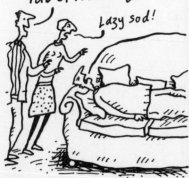

Lazy sod!

See also: HUSBANDS.

**HICCUPS** ~ A short-lived disease with no known cure. Wait patiently until the condition passes. There are various old wives' tales about keys, sipping water and frights but pay them no heed. In truth, hiccups are probably an alien language.

**HORNY** ~ Someone with horns, obviously.

**HUMILIATION** ~ Humiliate me!

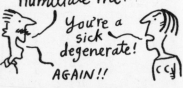

You're a sick degenerate!

AGAIN!!

**HUMP** ~ Having sex with someone with a hump. Some people, such as my friend, join specialist clubs to enjoy this sort of thing. Extraordinary!

# HUSBANDS~

## A PARASITE:

## PAWNING YOUR HUSBAND TO PAY HIS BILLS:

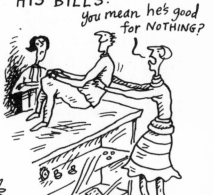

*you mean he's good for NOTHING?*

suck...

The <u>PROS & CONS</u> of vanishing husbands:

## THE PROS~
YOU CAN DRIVE THE CAR

*Wheee!*

## YOU DON'T HAVE TO KEEP PUTTING THE SEAT DOWN

*Floor's dry, too!*

## YOU GET CONTROL OF THE REMOTE

*No more sport!*

click!

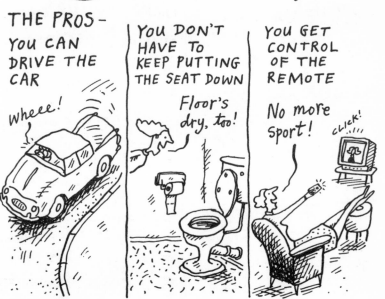

# H

NO BEARD HAIR IN THE WASH-BASIN

Spotless!

YOU GET THE WHOLE BED TO YOURSELF

AND no snoring!

THE CONS ~

Er... What cons?

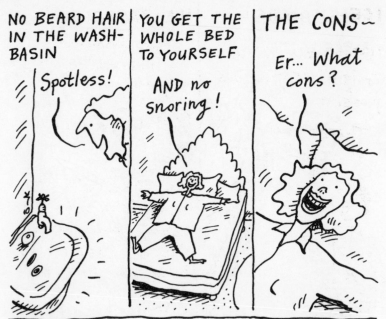

## HYGIENE ~

Hi, Jean!

Hiya, fellas!

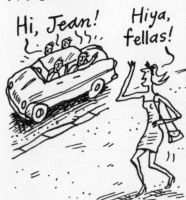

Keep yourself clean if you want good, clean fun, like Jean.

## HYPOCHONDRIAC ~
Gullible person who believes what their body is telling them.

## HYPOCRITE ~ Someone who asks you to do something they won't do themselves.

Do you love me?

YES!

Well, I don't love myself.

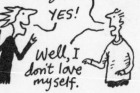

**ICE** ~ See FRIGID.

**IGNITE** ~ How to ignite someone's passion:

There's the blue touchpaper.

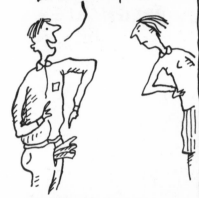

**IGNORE** ~
The more you ignore me, the more I want you!

Well, that's pretty futile, isn't it.

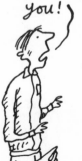

**ILL-BREEDING** ~ Your husband is ill-breeding again.

I'll KILL him!

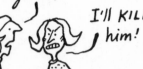

**ILLITERATE** ~ I see no point in writing about this problem as illiterate people won't be able to read it.

**IMMENSE** ~ A measurement of penis size. See also: PENIS.

**IMMUNE** ~ Chloe is immune to Roger's charms. See: BELOW.

**IMMUNIZED** ~
I'm immunized against them.

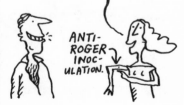

ANTI-ROGER INOCULATION.

# I

## IMPENETRABLE ~

*You're impenetrable, darling!*

## IMPOSTER ~

*Just a minute! You're not my husband!*

*And you're not my wife!*

## IMPOTENCE ~ The

mere mention of this magic word is enough to cause man's best friend to shrink, whimpering, back into his kennel. Even just <u>thinking</u> of the word will deflate a penis and it's owner in

less time than it takes to say "Don't you find me attractive?" or "Are you gay/straight?" *

* Delete according to which sex you are having sex with.

## IMPREGNABLE ~

*You're IMPREGNABLE, darling.*

*I hope so.*

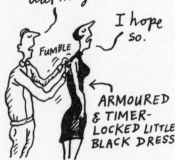

FUMBLE

ARMOURED & TIMER-LOCKED LITTLE BLACK DRESS

## IMPROMPTU ~

*I'm undressing!*

*That's IMPROPER, not 'impromptu'!*

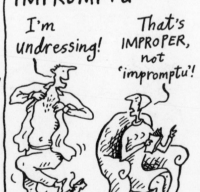

# INABILITY TO REMEMBER FACES ~

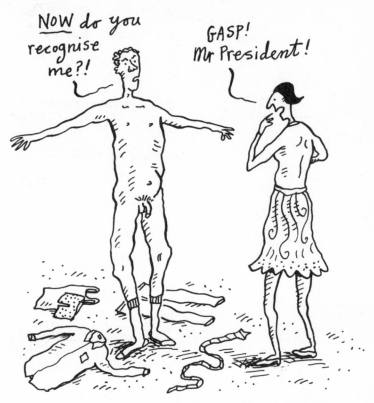

## IN-BREEDING ~

Breeding inside, as opposed to having sex out under the stars.

See also: INHIBITIONS.

## INCAPABLE ~

He's drunk!

He's incapable when he's NOT drunk, too.

# I

## INCONTINENT ~

Oh, you've been on the continent, Auntie?

No.

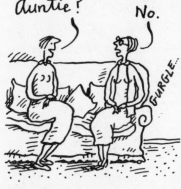

GURGLE...

## INCREDIBLE ~

Another measurement of penis size.

## INDECISIVE ~

Shall I be decisive or indecisive today...

## IN DENIAL ~ Of

COURSE you've got problems! Being in this state of denial is merely the thin lid barely keeping closed the heaving cauldron brim-full of your faults, mistakes, physical deformities and personal failings!! Thank GOD some good Samaritan gave you this book! (In your present state of mind I can't imagine that you actually BOUGHT it yourself.) With luck there is still time and you can be saved!

See also: DELUDING YOURSELF.

**INFERIORITY COMPLEX** ~ Perhaps you suffer from this because you really ARE inferior to most of your friends and work colleagues. Why not improve your status and self-esteem by purchasing one of these impressive degrees from the UNIVERSITY OF STEVEN APPLEBY!

BACHELOR OF BALLOON MODELLING

Voilà!

SPINSTER OF ORGANISED SITTING

You sit here... and Norman, you sit next to Irene...

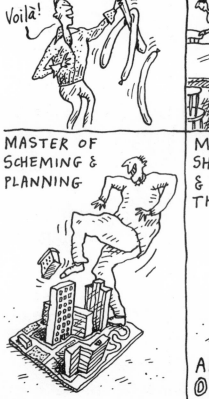

MASTER OF SCHEMING & PLANNING

MISTRESS OF SHALLOW & DEEP THINKING

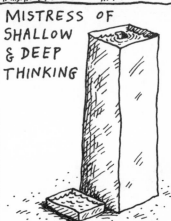

ALL ON **SPECIAL OFFER** THIS WEEK!

# I

## INHIBITIONS ~
The result of too much in-breeding. People who like to breed inside with the lights out will NEVER understand the pure animal elation of being stark naked on London Bridge having passionate sex with your loved one.

## IN-LAWS — see FAMILY.

## INSECTS IN THE BATH ~
An ugly situation. Just scoop them out and flush them down the toilet. Unless they turn out to be members of the family.

See also: TURNING INTO A GIANT INSECT.

## INSIGHT ~
Too much of this and you'll NEVER find a partner.

## INSOMNIA ~
Insomnia is a good way of avoiding dreams and nightmares while also giving you time to catch up on some of that thinking you didn't get finished during the day.

WILL I GET THE SACK TOMORROW?

ONE DAY I'M GOING TO DIE...

HOW CAN I PAY ALL THE BILLS?

EVERYTHING IS MY FAULT!

WHY DO I EXIST?

I'VE FORGOTTEN TO... SOMETHING!

## INSTABILITY ~

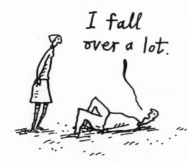

I fall over a lot.

## INTEREST ~

We all take an interest in rich and famous people. Although, of course, showing interest in them does not mean that they are interesting.

## INTOLERANCE ~

I am COMPLETELY intolerant of intolerance! I can't stand it! Just take a look at these NORMAL / ODD / UNUSUAL* examples of human behaviour and judge for yourselves.

I'm a potato!

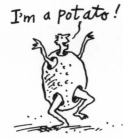

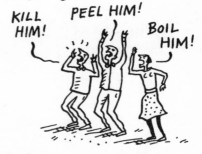

KILL HIM!

PEEL HIM!

BOIL HIM!

I'm a piece of cheese!

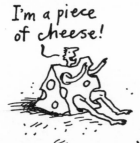

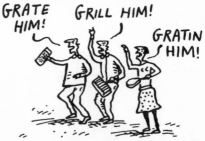

GRATE HIM!

GRILL HIM!

GRATIN HIM!

* DELETE ACCORDING TO YOUR PREJUDICES.

# I

## INTROVERT ~
Someone who looks inside themselves.

It's dark...

## INTUITION ~

You're cheating on me!

But you couldn't know...

I do NOW!!

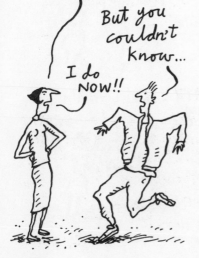

## INVERTEBRATE ~

You're spineless!

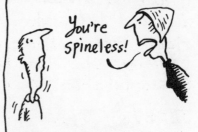

## IRRATIONAL ~

The car's broken down - let's kill some frogs!

## ITCHING ~ An ancient Chinese system of predicting the future based on wearing a woolly jumper and plotting the places you scratch on a chart. Infallible. It foretold the coming of this book.

**JEALOUSY** ~ Totally irrational anger directed at people richer, prettier, thiner, cleverer and more successful than you.

**JERSEY** ~ Small woolly island off the coast of France. Knitted in 1923.

**JINX** ~ Live the life of a hermit if you are one of these. In particular keep away from planes, trains, lottery contestants and, of course, me.

**JUMPING** ~ The best way to get from A to B if you are a superhero. Flying is too fast and tiring. Running like the wind can dry out the skin. Jumping is fun and impressive. It may also be used in dreams and animated cartoons.

See also: EXERCISE; TRAFFIC.

**JUVENILE DELINQUENT** ~ You'll grow out of it.

See also: AGEING. FORTY.

**KINKY** ~ Treat as a gift, not a problem, and you'll find surprise moments of pleasure around every corner! I recommend sieves, saucepans & the iron.

**KITCHEN** ~ Ideal room in which to indulge in kinky sex. Contains everything INCLUDING the kitchen sink!

Have fun!

# K

## KNEES

Why are so many people embarrassed by their knees? Because they are a sexy part of the body, of course – just like breasts, bottoms and bellies. So show them off!

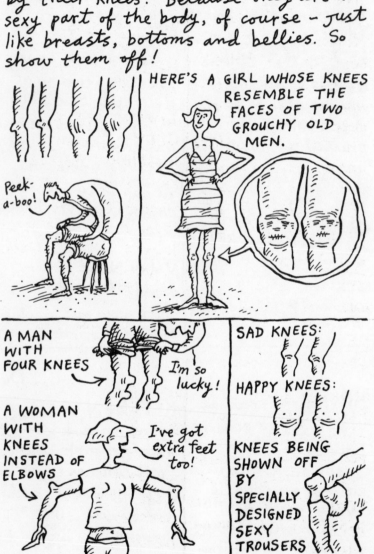

Peek-a-boo!

HERE'S A GIRL WHOSE KNEES RESEMBLE THE FACES OF TWO GROUCHY OLD MEN.

A MAN WITH FOUR KNEES → I'm so lucky!

A WOMAN WITH KNEES INSTEAD OF ELBOWS → I've got extra feet too!

SAD KNEES:

HAPPY KNEES:

KNEES BEING SHOWN OFF BY SPECIALLY DESIGNED SEXY TROUSERS

## LAUGHTER LINES ~

These are a real give away as to your great age. Nowadays it is cool to look sullen and straight-faced which means noone over the age of thirty has laughter lines. Fill them with wrinkle filler - sets to a smooth, sandable finish. And don't smile.

LAUGHTER LINES   WRINKLES

## LASTING ~ See: PREMATURE EJACULATION.

## LAZY ~ See: BED; GETTING UP; EXERCISE.

## LIKING RICE PUDDING ~ Now, this REALLY IS a perversion! Throw the devilish desert from Hell away THIS INSTANT and bring me jelly.

## LIVING IN THE COUNTRY ~ Quiet, peaceful, everyone is friendly and knows your business. For city lovers this is Hell. Move back to the city.

## LIVING IN THE CITY ~ Noisy, bustling, noone knows who you are and couldn't care less. For country lovers this is Hell. Move back to the country.

## LOCKED IN THE LAVATORY ~ Just like in that eerily perceptive song. In fact, why not sing the song as loudly as you can. Maybe someone will hear you...

HELP!

# L

## LONGEVITY ~ Here are some of the secrets of the well-preserved...

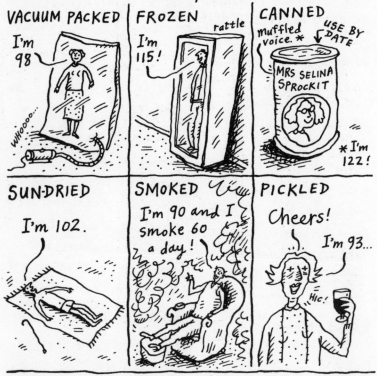

**VACUUM PACKED**
I'm 98
Whoooo

**FROZEN**
I'm 115!
rattle

**CANNED**
muffled voice. *
USE BY DATE
MRS SELINA SPROCKIT
* I'm 122!

**SUN-DRIED**
I'm 102.

**SMOKED**
I'm 90 and I smoke 60 a day!

**PICKLED**
Cheers!
I'm 93...
Hic!

**LOOKING IN OTHER PEOPLE'S DRAWERS AND CUPBOARDS ~** If a friend of yours comes into your home and starts to idly rummage through your drawers and cupboards, you are quite within your rights as a citizen to kill them. I'm sure I read that somewhere recently.

**LOST THINGS ~** Just think of the hours we waste looking for lost things like scissors, for example. Here's why:

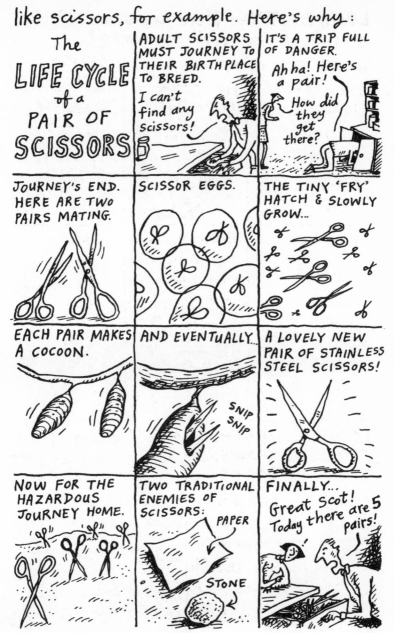

The
# LIFE CYCLE
of a
PAIR OF
SCISSORS

ADULT SCISSORS MUST JOURNEY TO THEIR BIRTHPLACE TO BREED.

I can't find any scissors!

IT'S A TRIP FULL OF DANGER.

Ah ha! Here's a pair!

How did they get there?

JOURNEY'S END. HERE ARE TWO PAIRS MATING.

SCISSOR EGGS.

THE TINY 'FRY' HATCH & SLOWLY GROW...

EACH PAIR MAKES A COCOON.

AND EVENTUALLY...

SNIP SNIP

A LOVELY NEW PAIR OF STAINLESS STEEL SCISSORS!

NOW FOR THE HAZARDOUS JOURNEY HOME.

TWO TRADITIONAL ENEMIES OF SCISSORS:

PAPER

STONE

FINALLY...

Great Scot! Today there are 5 pairs!

# L

**LOST YOUR WAY** ~ It's very easy to lose your way in life. If you're not careful you can lose sight of your goals, forget where you came from and where you're heading next. In no time at all you're trying to go up a one-way street the wrong way, horns are blaring, it's impossible to make a decision... Unless you have a LIFE COMPASS. Here's the one I bought with my pocket money in 1964:

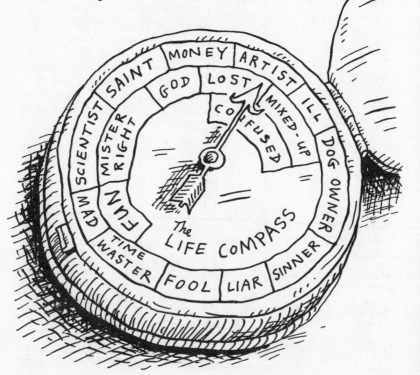

# L

I bought my Life Compass at a little shop called WINNIE'S. It never closes & is very hard to find. You have to search with your eyes shut.

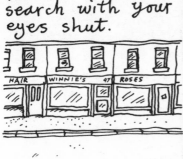

WINNIE'S also sells LIFE MAPS.

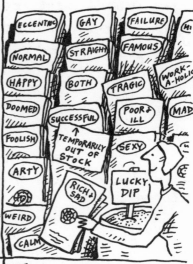

HERE'S MINE: =

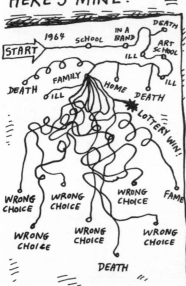

There are message balloons to buy too, as a kind of consolation if you can't find the right map.

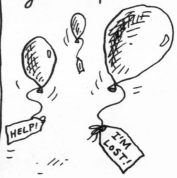

# L

**LOTTERY** ~ Don't deceive yourselves! You won't win. I will. See: LIFE MAP, previous page.

**LOVE** ~ When this happens the animal part of us has cut in and is setting our mating system in motion. Hormones zoom about triggering chemical reactions in the brain, secretions from the glands and crucial organs.

I'm in LOVE!

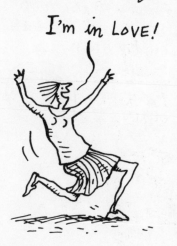

**LUGUBRIOUSNESS** ~ There's no such thing as love.

**LUST** ~ A similar feeling to love. Your stomach flips, you shiver, sweat and feel ill as your hormones and chemicals go crazy. Triggered by whatever you are attracted to – person, new car or pair of shoes – the effect is brief and culminates in orgasm or boredom. Love lasts a bit longer – hopefully.

I'm in LUST! Again...

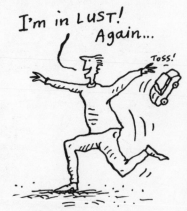

TOSS!

**LYING** ~ We all tell innocuous little fibs...

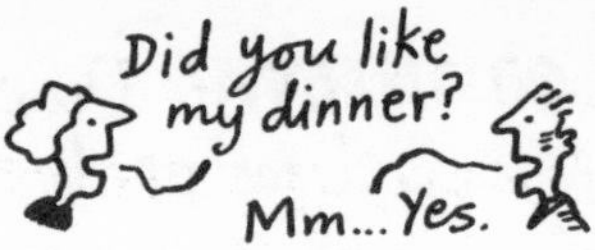


But some of us move on to tell more serious lies...

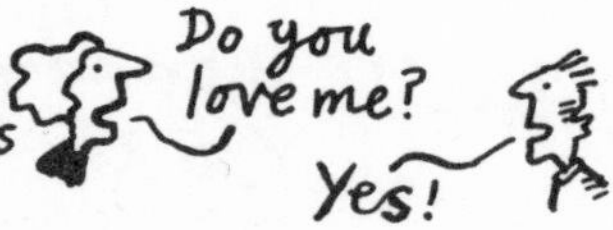


However, it isn't always easy to tell a lie from the truth.

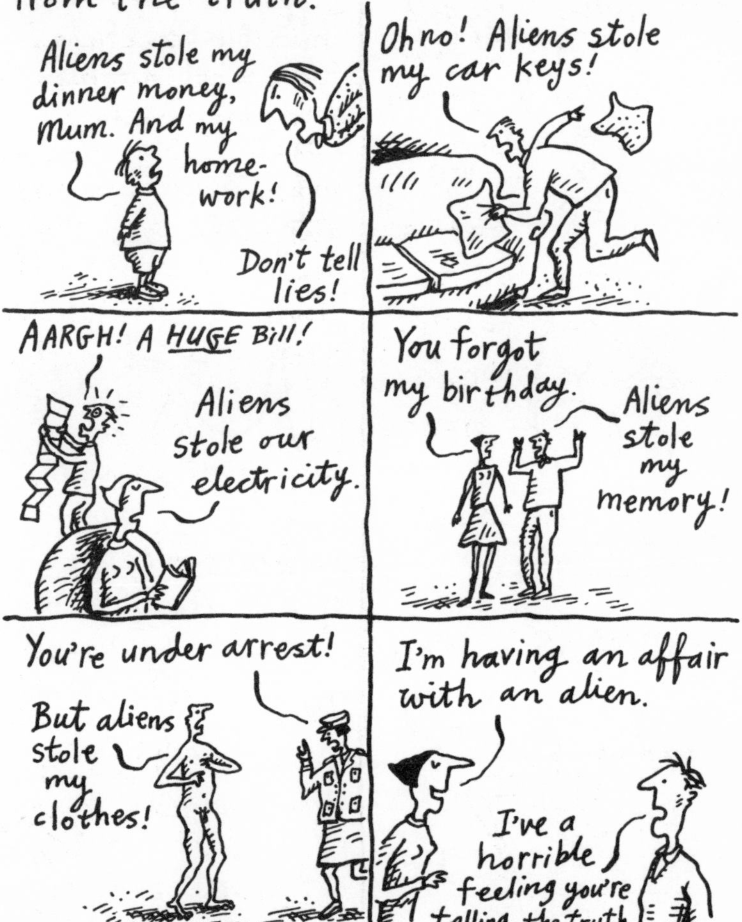

# M

## MACHISMO ~
Masculine pride.
Here's a macho
transvestite:

HEY!! Whaddiya
think YOU'RE
lookin' at,
JIMMY!?!

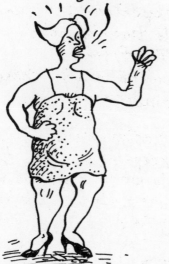

## MADNESS ~ When
the voices in my
head gather to
perform plays
during the day.

See also: DREAMS.

## MAN'S WORST FRIEND ~ Has to
be Doug Fairdale's
monstrously smug
Airedale.

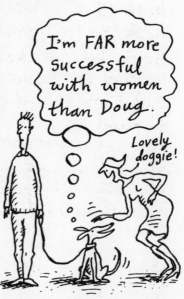

I'm FAR more
successful
with women
than Doug.

Lovely
doggie!

SOME OTHER THOUGHTS
OF DOUG'S AIREDALE:
'I can't stand being
TOUCHED by Doug.'
'Doug smells terrible.'
'Doug's voice irritates me.'
'Doug is boring.'
'I wish I lived with
ANYONE rather
than Doug.'

**MARIJUANA** — Plant of the hemp family containing cannabin. Due to a serious error in the binding of this book, pages 46-48 have been soaked in this resinous substance and should on no account be shredded and rolled into cigarettes to obtain a mellow and long-lasting high.

**MARRIAGE** — A blissful, mellow state similar to that obtained by smoking marijuana.

**MASTURBATION** — Sex without a partner. The rumour, that masturbation makes you go blind, was spread by unscrupulous oculists to encourage lucrative panic eye-testing. In fact my personal research suggests that masturbation prolongs youthfulness and extends life expectancy by up to twenty years. My friend corroborates these findings.

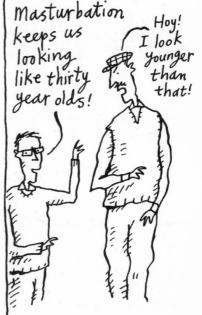

Masturbation keeps us looking like thirty year olds!

Hoy! I look younger than that!

# M

## MATRICIDE ~
Killing your mattress. An expensive problem, but not as bad as PATRICIDE - killing your patio. A new patio will set you back a small fortune.

## MEANING ~
My life has no meaning!

That's because you're not alive. You're just a drawing.

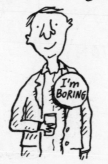

## MEANNESS -
Being sensible with money.

## MEETING SIMILAR PEOPLE ~
For those of you who despair of ever meeting a like-minded person to talk to or have sex with, worry no longer. Simply cut out the badge that describes you (or fill in one of the blanks) and pin it on. Next, watch out for someone wearing the same badge as you and Bob's your uncle! You're compatible!

[IF BOB _IS_ YOUR UNCLE, see also: HAVING AN UNFORTUNATE NAME]

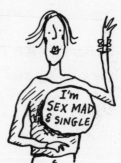

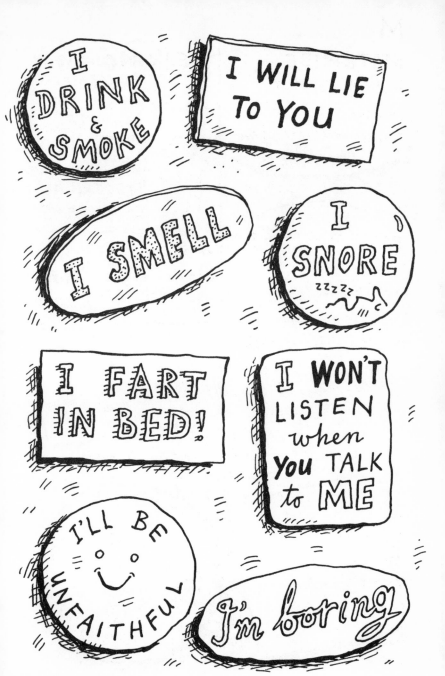

111

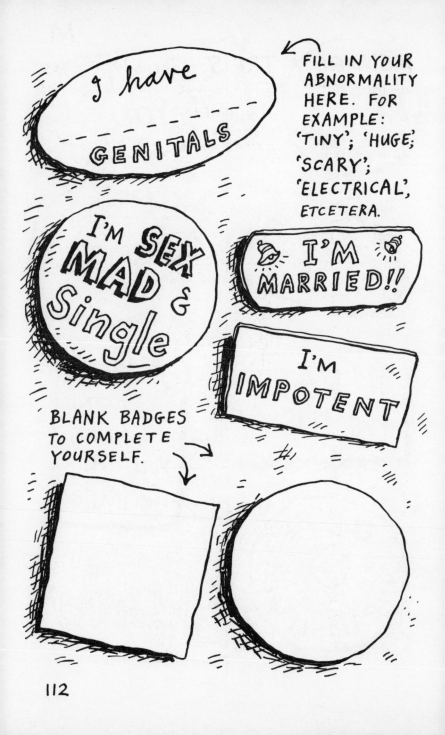

112

# MÉNAGE À TROIS — The advantages of multiple living arrangements are clear!

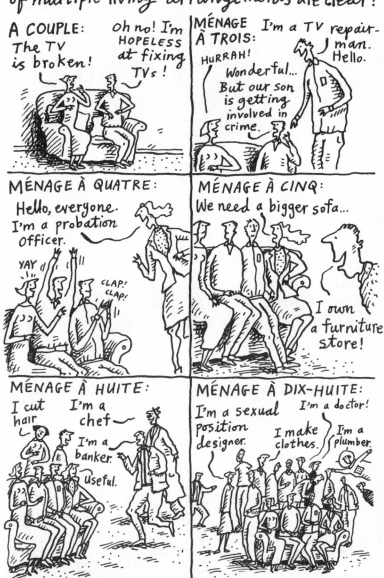

# M

## MENOPAUSE ~
A very long PMT.

## MENSTRUATION ~

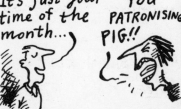

It's just your time of the month...

You PATRONISING PIG!!

## MIRROR ~

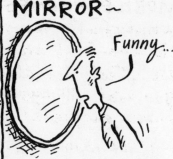

Funny...

See also: VAMPIRISM.

---

## MISSING SOCKS ~ Noone can ever find a pair of socks...

Mine are all exactly the same so I marked them with letters (A1 & A2, B1 & B2, etcetera) to help me tell each pair apart!

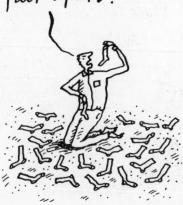

I can never find a matching pair of tights...

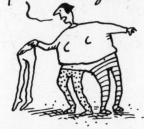

And I can never find an eight of socks!

**MOBILE PHONES** ～ Aren't they wonderful? You can be contacted in the event of an emergency, or for an utterly trivial reason, wherever you are! Always remember your mobile phone etiquette!

**i - SPEAK LOUDLY SO THE PERSON YOU'RE PHONING CAN HEAR YOU.**

HAW! HAW! HAW! Very GOOD, BRIAN!

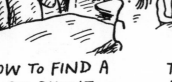

**ii - ALWAYS ANSWER!**

WRONG

I'll ignore my phone. YOU'RE more important!

BEEP!

RIGHT

Will you marry me...

Ssh! My phone's ringing!

BEEP!

**HOW TO FIND A LOST PHONE:**

I'll phone it up and listen for it ringing...

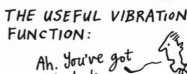

**THE USEFUL VIBRATION FUNCTION:**

Ah. You've got it, darling...

PREEP PREEP PREEP PREEP PREEP

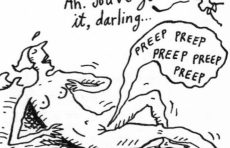

# M

## MOLE, GEORGE ~

Brilliant, eccentric humorist blackmailed into enforced encyclopedia compilation by a ruthless cartoonist. Mole was rumoured to have used an axe to dismember three of his second cousins but they were never found (and they never will be).

See also: FRIEND.

## MORNING SICKNESS ~

Congratulations! You're pregnant. If you are a man, you may be making medical history.

## MORTGAGE ~

Complex long-term financial commitment. In lay terms, imagine that you (and thousands of others) are on the end of a long leash held by a vast ogre with slavering jaws. You'll be eaten if you fall behind with your payments.

## MOTHER-IN-LAW ~

See: FAMILY.

## MUTANT ~ What we

all are compared to our distant grandparents, the slime creatures.

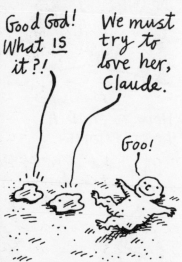

Good God! What IS it?!

We must try to love her, Claude.

Goo!

## MUTTON DRESSED AS LAMB ~ A sheep in a mini-skirt.

**NAG** ~ Repeatedly ask someone to do something, such as homework, without success. Eventually go blue in the face and send them to boarding school.

**NEIGHBOURS** ~ Everybody needs good neighbours. In the city this means you nod to each other in the street having forgotten one another's names. In the country you have an affair.

**NIGHTMARES** ~ Rather frightening premonitions. You wake up drenched in cold sweat, heart pounding, and think 'Phew! It was only a dream!' BE WARNED! It was NOT! During a nightmare you slip out of our world into one of many billion appalling variations on our reality which exist in parallel with our own. In no time at all you are being chased through quicksand by monsters or falling down, down, down through surreal versions of your childhood home. When you return to our reality (perceived as

Phew!

'waking up') turn the light
on quickly and check the
room thoroughly. Often
the inter-world doorway
has remained open long
enough for some 'thing' to
slip through. Usually just a few
flies, or perhaps a vampire zombie bat.
But best check under the bed just to
be sure. In America most citizens
keep a loaded firearm under the
pillow to combat evil. And who can
say they're not right?

AAARGH!!

I'm your
husband.

I
know!

---

NIPPLES — A
dangerous body part
best left covered
up. It is rumoured
that the poet Shelley
died of an over-
exposure to breasts.

SHELLEY'S
NIPPLES

OTHER
NIPPLES

NO MILK IN THE
HOUSE AFTER THE
SHOPS HAVE SHUT
~ A disaster. Always
check the fridge
before going to bed.
Even better, place
a regular order
with a nocturnal
milkman, who will
deliver last thing
at night instead of
in the morning.
Now, sleep easily.

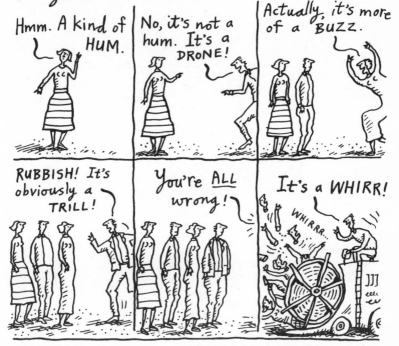

**NOISE** ~ Noise annoys, to quote the poet Shelley, so it's a marvellous thing to do when someone gets on your nerves.

Hmm. A kind of HUM.

No, it's not a hum. It's a DRONE!

Actually, it's more of a BUZZ.

RUBBISH! It's obviously a TRILL!

You're ALL wrong!

It's a WHIRR!

WHIRR...

**NON-SMOKER** ~ Someone who persecutes smokers.

**NOSE** ~ The organ through which we smell things like whether someone is smoking or not. Ugh. Their clothes stink! And their houses! Poo!! Have your nose surgically altered to look as pleasing as possible.

# N

Few noses are perfect, and even a perfect nose can be improved. Take a look at the pictures, below, where different noses have been placed on the same face to help you make a comparison. Once you've chosen your favourite, call Doctor Bob on FREE-PHONE NOSE (calls cost one pound per minute) for a consultation.

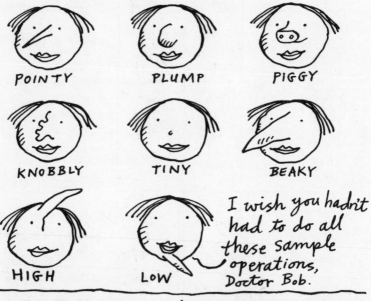

POINTY          PLUMP          PIGGY

KNOBBLY          TINY          BEAKY

HIGH          LOW

I wish you hadn't had to do all these sample operations, Doctor Bob.

**NOSE-PICKING ~** Choosing a new nose from the surgeon's catalogue.

**NUDISM ~** The strange, unnatural compulsion to take off your clothes.

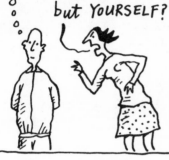

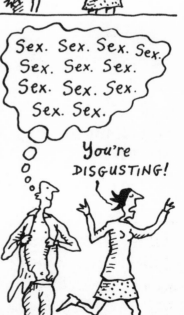

# O

**OCTOPUS** ~ See SOCKS.

**OEDIPUS COMPLEX** ~

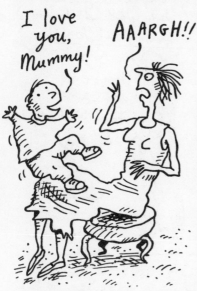

I love you, Mummy!

AAARGH!!

**OFFICE** ~ A place where grown-ups go, talk to their friends and come home grumpy.
See also: GRUMPY.

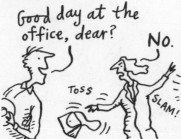

Good day at the office, dear?

NO.

TOSS

SLAM!

**ONE-TRACK MIND** ~ One of the secrets of success and true happiness. There's no room for doubt in a one-track mind. People with one-track minds just keep on and on at something until they become a professor, a captain of industry or even Prime Minister.

I've got a one-track mind. I can only think of you!

And I can only think of you, darling!

These two lovers have a very blissful but short life ahead. They have no space left in their minds for thoughts of eating.

# ONE-UP MAN SHIP

I have a penis the size of an elephant!

Well, I have an elephant the size of your penis.

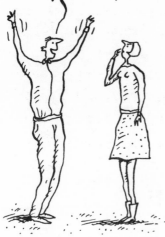

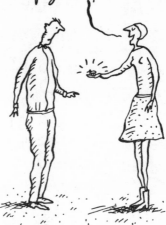

Aw... Isn't he cute.

SHE.

TOOT!

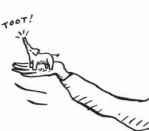

See also: PENIS SIZE; UNEXPECTED GUESTS.

**ONIONS** – A very sad and tragic vegetable whose short life leads only to death and dismemberment.

Boo hoo! Boo hoo!

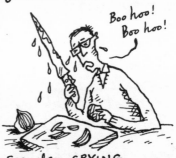

See also: CRYING.

# O

**OPTIMISM** ~ The only thing which keeps onions going.

**ORAL SEX** ~ Talking about sex instead of doing it.
See also: TALKING TOO MUCH.

**ORGANS, VITAL** ~ I have tried donating my organs after death but nobody wants them. The whole is rejected in life & I am rejected piecemeal after death.
See also: UNPOPULARITY.

**OSTRACIZE** ~ see: UNPOPULARITY.

**OSTRICH COMPLEX** ~ A useful defence against attack by thugs. A bit like learning Karate or Judo, but easier. Simply take a bucket of sand with you at all times.
WHAT TO DO:

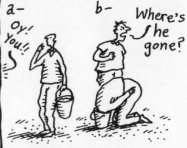

a-
Oy! You!!

b-
Where's he gone?

**OVER, IT'S** ~

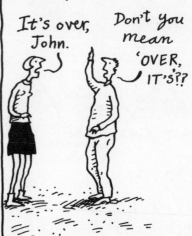

It's over, John.

Don't you mean 'OVER, IT'S'??

**OVERDRAFT** ~ When my bank says 'It's over, Steven.'

124

## PANIC ATTACKS ~
An attack by desperate headless chicken people who are slowly starving to death. Sit quietly, breathe deeply, count to ten and it will go away.

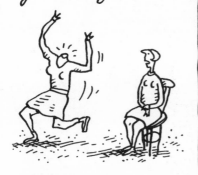

## PARANOIA ~
Ever felt like you are being watched? Well, it's true. <u>I'M</u> watching you! At all times! How else do you think I could learn all the things I have put into this book?

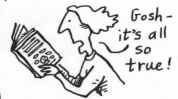

Gosh - it's all so true!

## PARASITES ~
See: HUSBANDS.

## PARENTS ~
See: FAMILY.

## PENIS ~
The male Staff of Office. Useful for peeing out of and, ahem, in the bedroom, but aside from that its main function is as an organ which proves problematic in the tailoring of tight trousers. Until now! I have discovered that the penis makes an excellent barometer. Simply tattoo the markings around

**P**

your groin, as I have done. Or make
use of the diagram below.

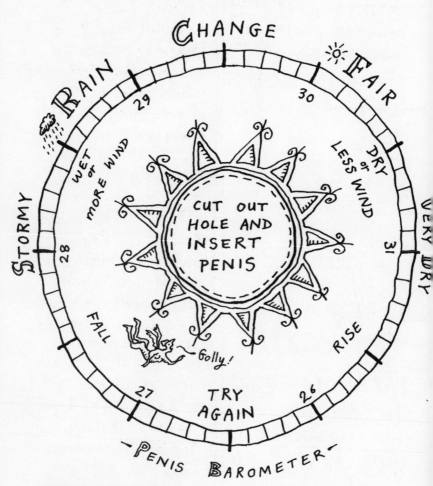

HOW TO USE:
Tap penis lightly a couple of times.
Wait a moment until it settles.
Take reading.

## Measurement scale (left column)

YAHOO! — 7

CRIKEY! — 6

AVERAGE — 5

MEDIUM — 4

SMALL — 3

HMM... — 2

WHERE IS IT? — 1

OFF THE SCALE - YOU SHOULD BE PICKLED IN A JAR AFTER DEATH FOR ALL TO GAWP AT!

# P

# PENIS SIZE —

Size DOES matter. It has been established that there is a clear correlation between penis size and depression (in both men and women). So look happy.

HOW TO USE THE MEASURE:

Place your penis into the fold in the centre of the book.

Hmm. Quite sexy...

NOTE - In the interest of male self-esteem the inches, left, have been made slightly smaller than usual.

# P

## PHOBIAS

PHOBIAS ~ This vast subject is too huge to go into in depth (FEAR OF TAKING ON SOMETHING TOO BIG), so I intend to devote an entire book to it in the near future. Probably. (FEAR OF COMMITMENT). The Classic Phobias, such as fear of spiders, open spaces, confined spaces and so on, usually make sound sense when you examine them. Who in their right mind likes spiders? And no one wants to be shut into a cupboard or trapped in a lift with other people's children. However,

← FEAR OF THIS BOOK

modern life has generated some new, sensible phobias to watch out for...

FEAR OF ANSWERING MACHINES:
It's got 87 messages on it!

FEAR OF TOASTERS:
It can't see me down here!

FEAR OF PHONING:
Hello? Mum! Thank God...

FEAR OF CLOTHING:
Wait! I'll undress!

FEAR OF BEING FOUND OUT:
I'm no good at my job! I'm out of my depth!

And, of course, FEAR OF YOUR OWN GENE CODE (why you have phobias) and FEAR OF CATCHING A PHOBIA.

# PIERCING ~

Everyone is into body decoration nowadays. Here's a man who's just had something-or-other pierced and a woman who's got this-or-that pierced.

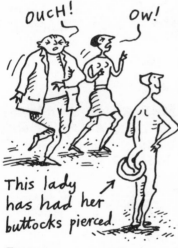

OUCH!

Ow!

This lady has had her buttocks pierced.

# PIGEON-TOED ~

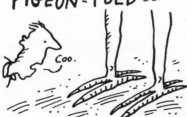

Coo.

# PILES ~

Piles of money? Piles of friends? Or just piles. It makes a big difference. If the latter, then <u>DON'T</u> talk about them! People are repulsed. Piles of money, on the other hand, is seen as attractive and you'll soon have piles of friends.

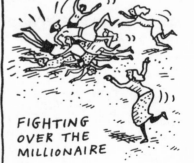

FIGHTING OVER THE MILLIONAIRE

My friend once had piles of friends, until he had piles.

# PIMPLES — See: SPOTS.

# P

**PLAGUES** ~ The Ten Plagues of Christmas: Tinselitis, Groping, Scorning of the First Born, Indigestion, Flatulence, Locusts, Cheap Wine, Blood on the Pudding, Relations, Cat Urine, Boils and Lice on the Christmas Frog.

**PLANTS** ~ When the plants take over, which of us will be weeds?

**PLAYING THE MARTYR** ~

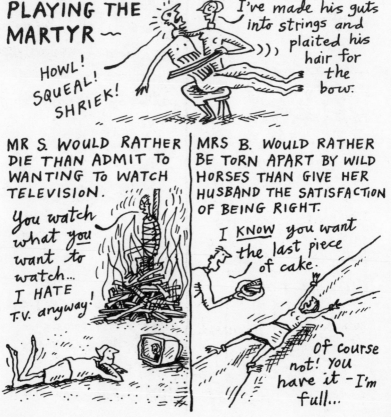

HOWL! SQUEAL! SHRIEK!

I've made his guts into strings and plaited his hair for the bow.

MR S. WOULD RATHER DIE THAN ADMIT TO WANTING TO WATCH TELEVISION.

You watch what you want to watch... I HATE T.V. anyway!

MRS B. WOULD RATHER BE TORN APART BY WILD HORSES THAN GIVE HER HUSBAND THE SATISFACTION OF BEING RIGHT.

I KNOW you want the last piece of cake.

Of course not! YOU have it - I'm full...

NAT WOULD RATHER BOIL SLOWLY IN OIL THAN MENTION HIS CAT ALLERGY.

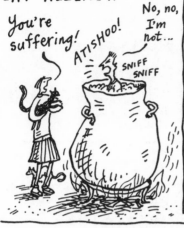

You're suffering!

ATISHOO!

SNIFF SNIFF

No, no, I'm not...

SEBASTIAN JUST CAN'T SAY SORRY, EVEN WHEN HE'S IN THE WRONG.

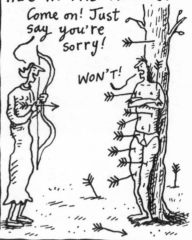

Come on! Just say you're sorry!

WON'T!

**POLITE** ~ Being polite costs nothing so it can't be worth doing, then.

**POPPYCOCK** ~ A load of bollocks, or a poppy cock. Either way, a SERIOUS personal problem. A load of balls are NOT a pretty sight in a tight pair of trousers:

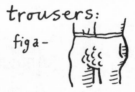

fig a –

While a poppy cock is good only for pollinating other poppies:

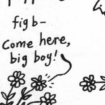

fig b –
Come here, big boy!

See a specialist.

# P

## PREMATURE EJACULATION ~

Pretty inconvenient if your ejaculation is so premature that it takes place earlier in the day or even the previous week.

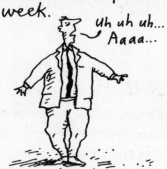

Uh uh uh... Aaaa...

Clever use of your diary and watches synchronised to the second SHOULD enable you to time sexual activity so that it matches an ejaculation from next week.

Uh uh. Aaah! That will be fantastic, darling!

With practise you'll be able to time sex to last a few hours before next Friday's ejaculation kicks in.

## PREMATURE TALKING ~

I'll have the fishcakes, followed by.... Oh. I'm not at the restaurant yet!

## PREMATURE ANSWERING ~

Yes! Yes! I WILL!!    But I haven't said anything yet!

## PRIDE ~

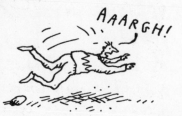

AAARGH!

## PROPOSAL ~

Will you marry me?

No. No. No. No. No.

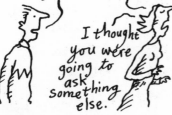

I thought you were going to ask something else.

## PRAYING MANTIS ~

Mrs Praying Mantis eats the head of Mr Praying Mantis while he is engaged in the act of love. I have been asked not to make any jokes about "giving head", so I won't.

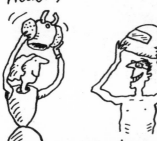

It's a good thing, because my wife likes to dress up as a praying mantis and I am forced to wear a motorcycle helmet.

## PSYCHOLOGICAL PROBLEMS ~ These

problems are all inside the mind.

DO I EXIST?

No.

Well, that's okay then, isn't it. Noone can see them like they can if you've got spots, hairy legs or an elephant's head. But CAN this problem be ignored? Some people believe that they've been born into the wrong body:

I'm a Venusian waffle-sexual. Isn't it obvious?

133

Others believe that more than one person lives inside them.

Whose turn is it to brush the teeth?

Not me!

I'm doing the chewing today.

Who are you?

A very egotistical person may believe that they are the centre of the universe. Another person might think the world revolves around someone else, such as the postman.

Particularly self-important people think that the world, and everything in it, exists only in their own minds.

I don't want to boast, but the truth is that recent research shows the universe to exist only in MY mind. The book you're reading doesn't exist outside my mind. Your house doesn't exist and YOU don't exist – unless I think of you. Ho hum. Time to think about something else...

**PULL YOUR SOCKS UP~** If your socks keep falling down just throw them away & buy a new pair.

**PULL YOURSELF TOGETHER ~** You might need the help of a friend. Make sure you don't discard any left-over body parts until everything is working properly.

THERE ARE
NO PROBLEMS
BEGINNING
WITH Q.

# R

**RADIANT** ~ Glowing from contact with radioactivity. Keep well clear of radiant people!

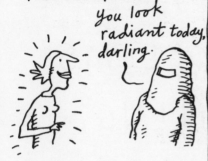

You look radiant today, darling.

**RAGE** ~ See ANGER.

**REALITY** ~ A much overrated state.

**RECTUM** ~ See ANUS.

**REGIONAL ACCENT** ~ See a speech therapist, buy gum.

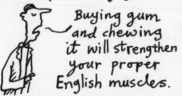

Buying gum and chewing it will strengthen your proper English muscles.

**REINCARNATION** ~ A problem if someone you don't like is reincarnated as something near you, such as your new cat, car, child, chair or coal bucket.

**REJECTION** ~ Not always a problem.

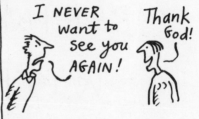

I NEVER want to see you AGAIN!

Thank God!

**RELATIVES** ~ See FAMILY.

**REPTILE** ~ Cold-blooded slimy man covered in scales. How on earth anyone could mistake a reptile for Mr Right is beyond me

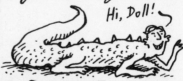

Hi, Doll!

**REPULSIVE** ~ See ABOVE.

# RETENTIVE ~

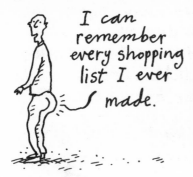

I can remember every shopping list I ever made.

# ROMANTIC ~

Being a romantic is always a problem. The world is a big bad place full of problems (see the rest of this book) and romanticising it is inaccurate. You're in for a let-down.

My knight in shining armour has turned out to be a male chauvenist pig!

WHERE'S MY DINNER!

# RUBBER ~

What I like to imagine you wearing as you read this book, crossing your shiny black thighs, little beads of sweat trickling from your wrists and ankles...

# RUBBISH ~

As in:

Stop watching that rubbish on T.V. - Come back to bed and service me, Gerald!

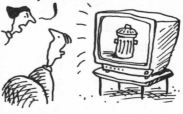

# RUNNY NOSE ~

An unfortunate problem with some of the cheaper plastic noses used in Doctor Bob's cosmetic surgery.

# S

**SACRIFICE** ~ You must make sacrifices in order to make a relationship work.

How about sacrificing the children?

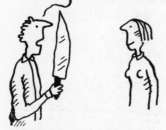

**SADISM** ~ Being cruel to be kind.

**SANTA/SATAN** ~ Both wear red, tempt children & have horned familiars.

**SAUCY** ~ Covered in chocolate sauce.

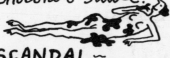

**SCANDAL** ~ That's scandalous! There are people starving in other countries!

**SCARS** ~ Attractive to some, but if you don't agree why not get your surgeon to be artistic in his or her cutting?

HERRING BONE SCAR:

PORTRAIT SCAR:

MOUNTAIN LANDSCAPE SCAR:

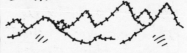

**SCROTUM** ~ Ugly and wizened little hairy bag. Men keep their valuables in one.

**SEANCE** ~ Hello... I didn't know you were dead, darling!

**SECOND COUSIN** ~ From the Greek "worthy of being struck repeatedly with an axe". See also: MOLE, G; FRIEND.

**SEX** ~ The act of reproduction between two, or preferably more, creatures.

**SEX WITH ALIENS** ~ The ultimate perversion. Where do you penetrate it? And with <u>what</u> does it penetrate you? According to abductees, alien flying saucers are filled by one huge circular mattress – and it ISN'T for protection against the G-force of take off!

Welcome aboard, mr Appleby...

**SELF-CATERING** ~ I make sandwiches...

**SELF-DESTRUCTIVE** ~ But I'm no good at it.

**SELF-EMPLOYED** ~ You're sacked!

**SELF-PITY** ~ I lost my job...

**SELF-RESPECT** ~ I've got none!

**SELL-BY DATE** ~ Time to kill myself.

**SHRIVEL** ~ See IMPOTENT.

**SHY** ~ my penis is a bit shy... No. It's shrivelled.

# S

## SICK BUILDINGS ～ They're bad for you!

A SLIGHTLY NAUSEOUS BUILDING. THIS ONE IS A CAR PARK.

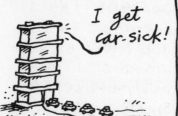

*I get car-sick!*

A BUILDING WITH A TEMPERATURE.

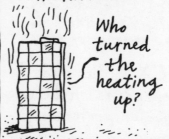

*Who turned the heating up?*

A HOLIDAY HOME SUFFERING FROM A HEADACHE.

*I can't stand the constant screaming of children.*

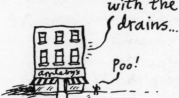

YOU'RE DEAD!

BUDDA BUDDA BUDDA... AWW!

A BUILDING WITH A FEVER.

*I need air conditioning!*

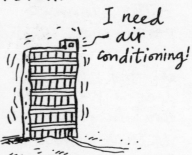

A CAFÉ WITH DIARRHOEA.

*There must be something wrong with the drains...*

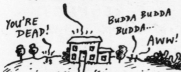

Poo!

THIS BUILDING HAS FAINTED.

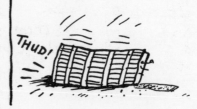

THUD!

**SINGING IN THE BATH** ~ Can be annoying.

Dad's gone very quiet...

He's DROWNED!

I drowned him!

**SISTER** — See FAMILY.

**SIZE** ~ See PENIS.

**SLEEPING LIKE A BABY** ~ A surprising number of grown-up men and women like to wear huge nappies, climb into giant cots and sleep like babies. And if it gives them a good night's sleep, then why not.

See also: INSOMNIA.

**SMELLING LIKE A CHEESE** ~ Everyone you meet looks at you strangely, am I right? That's because their mouths are watering. No amount of washing will remove the smell because you ARE a cheese.

Turn yourself in at the nearest cheese works.

**SMOKING** — Someone with a very tiny death wish. Of course, they will deny this.

**SNEEZING** — Used thoughts being expelled to make room for more. But remember – DON'T breathe in other people's old thoughts in case you catch sick ideas.

# SNORING —

SNORT! GRUNT! WHISTLE! HONK! TOOT! SNUFFLE!

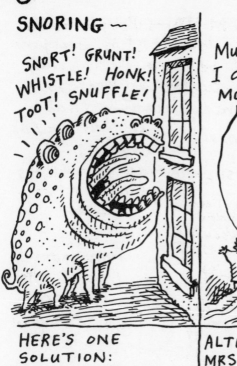

Mummy! Mummy! I can hear a MONSTER roaring!!

Don't be frightened, darling. It's only your father snoring.

SNORT! BELLOW!

HERE'S ONE SOLUTION:

a- SOUND-PROOF MASK.

b- PIPE FROM MASK TAKES NOISE TO BE JETTISONED HARMLESSLY OUTSIDE.

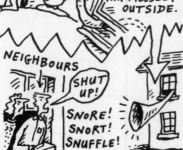

NEIGHBOURS

SHUT UP!

SNORE! SNORT! SNUFFLE! SQUEAK!

ALTERNATIVELY, TRY MRS APPLEBY'S FOOL-PROOF TIP TO SILENCE SNORING PERMANENTLY.

Hold a pillow over the snorer's face... like so...

I want to help, Mum!

UTTER SILENCE

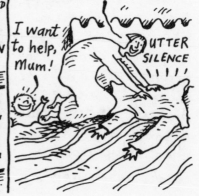

**SPEAKING YOUR MIND** — People who speak their minds see this as a virtue, but don't be fooled! Speaking your mind is actually a VERY serious personal problem!

HERE IS A PERSON SPEAKING HIS MIND:

You are not a nice person!

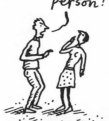

AND HERE IS THE SAD RESULT:

I feel AWFUL about myself now...

BUT WATCH WHAT HAPPENS IF <u>SHE</u> SPEAKS HER MIND BACK TO <u>HIM</u>.

You criticise me because YOU'VE got a problem! You're unhappy! You're mean!

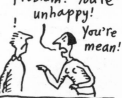

HE CAN'T TAKE HIS OWN MEDICINE!

WAAAA!! WAAAA!! WAAAAA!!

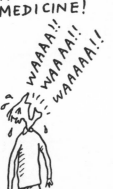

SO LET'S LEARN FROM THIS AND BE NICE & POLITE TO EACH OTHER.

You look GREAT!

You too!

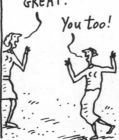

Silly cow.

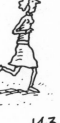

# S

## SPIRITUALITY – drinking spirits.

Vodka, whisky, gin, rum...

**INVISIBLE SPIRITS:**

Aargh! They've disappeared! Scary!!

You've drunk them all.

**CONTACTING THE SPIRITS:**

Simply turn over an empty glass... Yes, it's moving!

SQUEAK SQUEAK

**GHOSTS:**

CHOKE! I can feel an invisible SPIRIT HAND at my THROAT!!

You're suffering from DTs.

**DEMONS:**

I'm POSSESSED by SPIRITS!!

Yes, I can smell them on your breath.

I'm being HAUNTED!

By a sense of GUILT I hope! You've drunk all my spirits!

EMPTY

## SPIRITUALITY – ghosts.

Clouds are the ghosts of people who have died.

UGH! Ghosts are weeing on us!

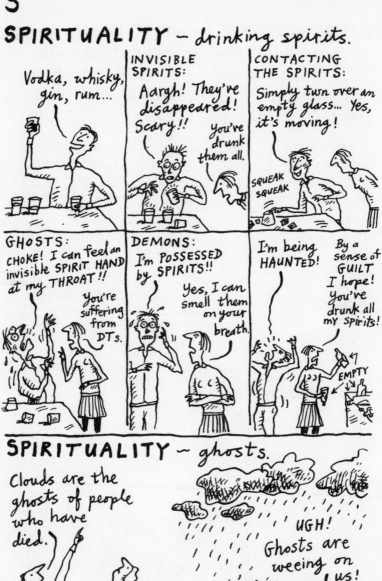

# SPIRITUALITY — *level of consciousness.*

It is generally a good thing to increase your level of spirituality — just make sure you don't lose touch with reality.

WRONG ⟶
Heightened spirituality isn't compatible with a desk job.

*I can't answer the phone!*

ME - JUST RIGHT!
Here I am getting the phone, work, money and other material rewards.

TREEP... TREEP...
TREEP...
TREEP...

WRONG ⟶
This man has reached a lower level of consciousness.

BELCH!!

# S

**SPOTS** — These secret storehouses of pus. These tiny roseate hillocks of angry flesh, these islands in a skinly sea sometimes rising to a tempting point are to be treasured by anyone over nineteen. They show that deep down we are still alive, vibrant teenagers. May they never leave us.

SOME SPOTS:

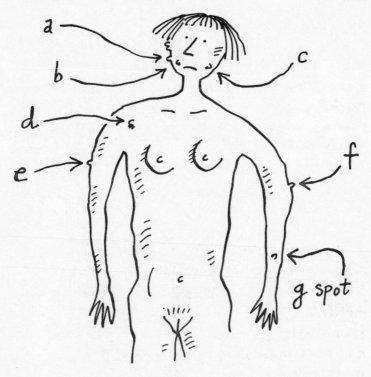

There are all kinds of different spots
of all sizes, colours and shapes.
Here are a few you may 'spot' on
yourself or a friend.

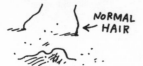

BLACKHEAD

WHITEHEAD

A SPOT WITH A
HEAD ON IT

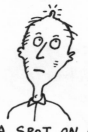

←— NORMAL
HAIR

AN INGROWING
HAIR

AN INGROWING
HAIRSTYLE

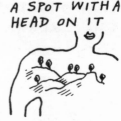

A BEAUTY
SPOT

A SPOT ON A
PERSON

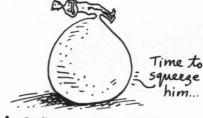

Time to
squeeze
him...

A PERSON ON A SPOT

I think that spots are a
communication from beyond the
grave. A kind of code, or 'body brail',
which dead relatives use to get in
touch with the living. Over leaf are
some examples I received recently
from my mother (deceased).

SPOT COMMUNICATIONS

" I don't trust that man at the garage."

" You really must do more exercise!"

" Don't eat so much chocolate. It isn't good for you."

"And are you remembering to wear a vest?"

"Let me give you a word of advice on how to bring up your children"...

"Your father and I liked your last book – but how about doing one on death?"

**SEEING SPOTS —** Noticing spots on yourself or your friends. If you see spots of blood on your clothing, turn yourself in to the police and tell them where your three victims are hidden, Mole!
See also: MOLE; FRIEND.

**SOUL —** The immortal part of us which governs our conscience and makes us human. Can be sold, which most people appear to have done judging from the state of the world.

**STEALING —** This is against the law so don't do it. How would <u>you</u> feel if I came along and pinched your diamond-encrusted solid gold Rolex? Yes, exactly. So don't take mine! Even Robin Hood was technically breaking the law so don't justify yourself with that old argument.

**STOLEN THOUGHTS—**

Oh, er... What was I going to say?

Oh no! His thoughts have been... Er...

**STOMACH —** Flat, like a washboard. Or it's renamed 'belly'.

**SWEAT —** Evil-smelling ooze which seeps out through your skin. Try panting instead. It's more dignified.

149

# S

**SWOLLEN HEAD** ~ An unpleasant and unsightly disorder which will make you unpopular. No one likes a person with a swollen head. Luckily this problem is easily treated by a sympathetic G.P. or therapist.

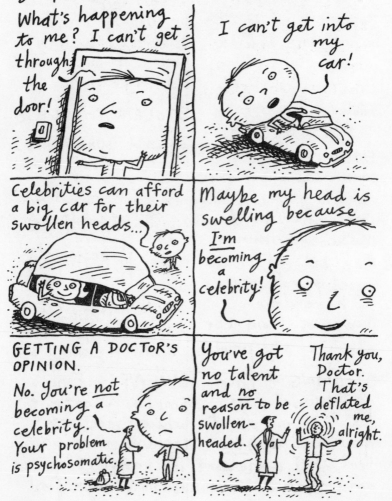

What's happening to me? I can't get through the door!

I can't get into my car!

Celebrities can afford a big car for their swollen heads...

Maybe my head is swelling because I'm becoming a celebrity!

GETTING A DOCTOR'S OPINION.

No. You're _not_ becoming a celebrity. Your problem is psychosomatic.

You've got _no_ talent and _no_ reason to be swollen-headed.

Thank you, Doctor. That's deflated me, alright.

## TACTLESSNESS —

Saying what you really think. Is it being truthful or being unpleasant? Either way the end result is usually that the person you're talking to is offended and won't have anything to do with you. Ever.

*I don't like you... Oops! That came out wrong!*

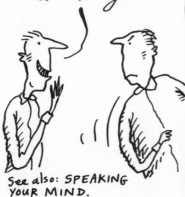

See also: SPEAKING YOUR MIND.

## TALKING ANIMALS —

*I've got a talking parrot - listen!*

*Hello!*

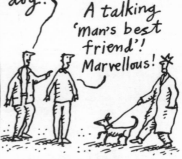

*Well, Bob's got a talking dog.*

*A talking 'man's best friend'! Marvellous!*

*He's certainly NOT my best friend! He told my wife I was having an affair.*

*Remember! I've got my eye on you...*

# T

## TALKING TO A CHILD — Some people have a problem with this. Here's how to do it.

**Fig a — WRONG!**
DON'T TALK <u>DOWN</u> TO HIM.

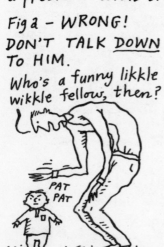

Who's a funny likkle wikkle fellow, then?

PAT PAT

**Fig b — RIGHT!**
TALK TO HIM ON HIS OWN LEVEL.

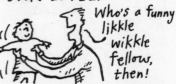

Who's a funny likkle wikkle fellow, then!

**Fig c — RIGHT AGAIN!**
Who's a funny likkle wikkle fellow, then!

---

## TALKING TOO MUCH —

When I said 'use your tongue' I didn't mean TALK!!

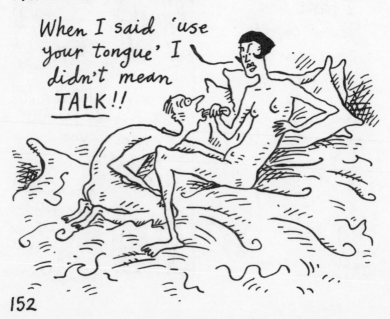

152

# T

**TASTE** ~ It is important to cultivate good taste, otherwise your taste horizons close in and your mind narrows.

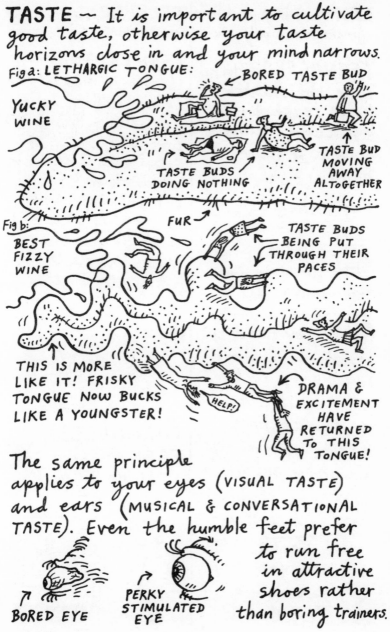

Fig a: LETHARGIC TONGUE:

YUCKY WINE

BORED TASTE BUD

TASTE BUD MOVING AWAY ALTOGETHER

TASTE BUDS DOING NOTHING

Fig b:

BEST FIZZY WINE

FUR

TASTE BUDS BEING PUT THROUGH THEIR PACES

THIS IS MORE LIKE IT! FRISKY TONGUE NOW BUCKS LIKE A YOUNGSTER!

HELP!

DRAMA & EXCITEMENT HAVE RETURNED TO THIS TONGUE!

The same principle applies to your eyes (VISUAL TASTE) and ears (MUSICAL & CONVERSATIONAL TASTE). Even the humble feet prefer to run free in attractive shoes rather than boring trainers.

BORED EYE

PERKY STIMULATED EYE

153

# T

**TAX** — A big problem if you can't pay it.

**TEENAGERS** — Hurrah! Once the children have reached this age they're almost ready to leave home.

**TEETHING** — Once you're a teenager you're past this little problem for a few years. Until you start dating, then you need to brush and floss regularly to keep your smile sweet and sparkling. Again, in old age you may suffer teething problems with your new false teeth. Don't kiss too vigorously.

*You've got my teeth too!*

**TELEPHONE** — See: PHOBIAS.

**TEMPERATURE** — Having a high temperature is usually nothing to worry about. If your small child is ill with a temperature take him or her into bed with you — they make marvellous hot-water bottles.

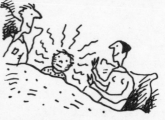

**THANKLESS TASK** —

*Living with you!*

154

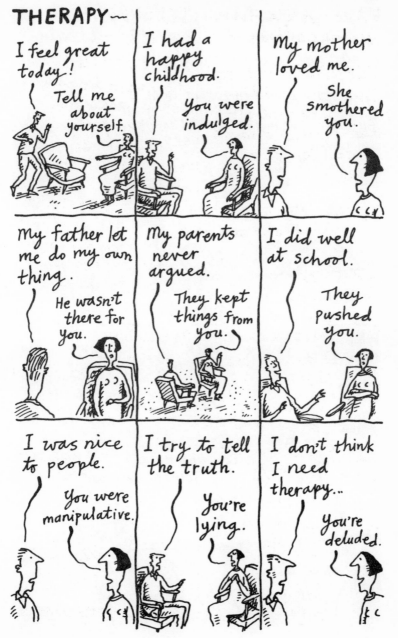

T

Have you noticed how people who are having therapy think it's suddenly okay to behave badly?

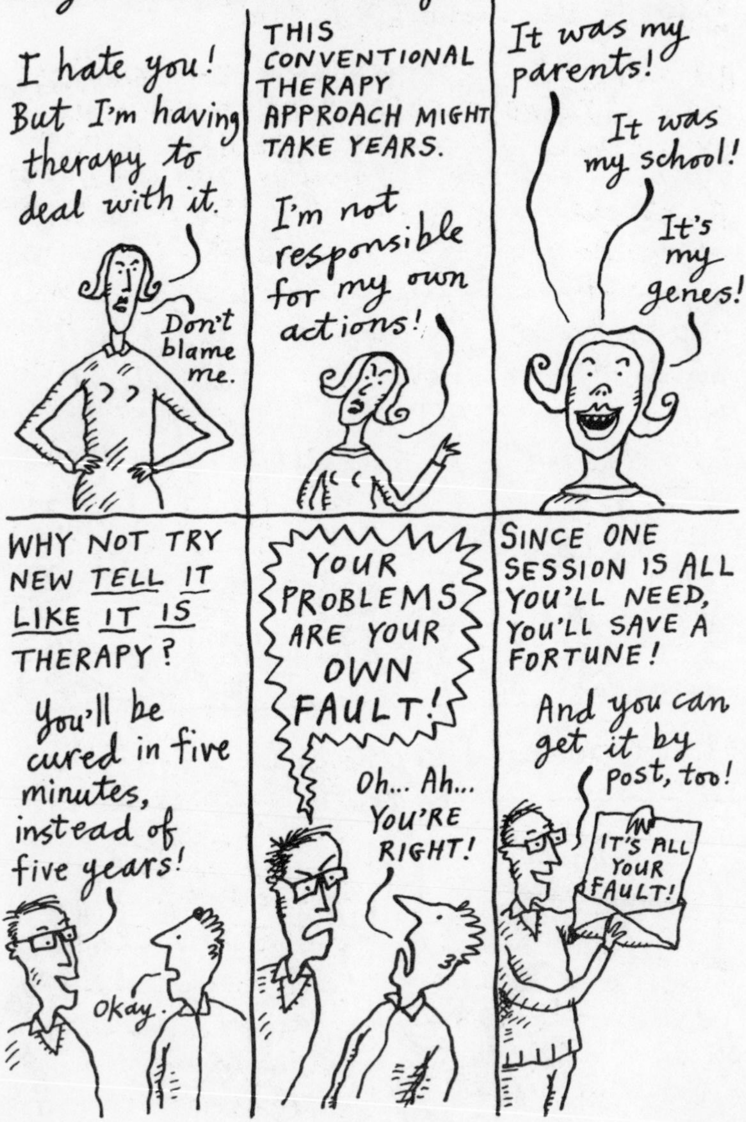

# THINKING YOU KNOW WHAT YOU'RE DOING ~ People with this problem are continually getting themselves into trouble. Because they don't.

**AN ENTIRE CITY IS FUSED BY A COW.**

The stupid thing has wired the plug up the wrong way round.

**ALL THE ELECTRICS IN A MAJOR HOTEL ARE BLOWN BY A HIPPO.**

Aren't animals dumb? Fancy watching TV in the bath!

**THE ENTIRE NATIONAL GRID IS PUT OUT OF ACTION BY A HERD OF BUFFALO.**

I _KNEW_ we shouldn't have employed them as repairmen...

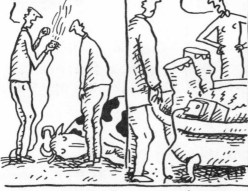

DANGER

# THINKING TOO MUCH ~

Why are we alive?

In order to get drunk! Come on!

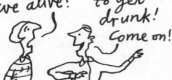

# THREESOME ~ A
sexual position. See also: MÉNAGE À TROIS.

# TIRED ~ Either
you've got children, or you're having too many threesomes.

# T

## TISSUE OF LIES ~

You've told me a tissue of lies, luckily. I was able to tear it apart in a few seconds!

## TONE ~ Are you looking this up because you want to tone up your body, or because you don't like the tone of this book? If the latter, then LOOK HERE! People with your sort of squalid little problem need HELP! So stop complaining and READ... And if it was body toning you were interested in then look up 'exercise'.

158

## TOUPEE ~ See BALDNESS.

## TRAFFIC ~ See OVERLEAF.

## TRAITOR ~

You've betrayed me!

What are you going to do about it?!

Have you executed!

## TRUST ~ A cereal bowl can be glued back together, but trust, once broken, cannot be repaired.

Forgive me...

NO!

Telling the truth is important — admit to breaking the bowl.
See also: TRUTH.

## TRYING TOO HARD ~ Very suspicious.

**TRAFFIC** ~ This is a problem which will get worse and worse. Here is a glimpse of the future. A future in which cars, people carriers and small vans feast on a pedestrian.

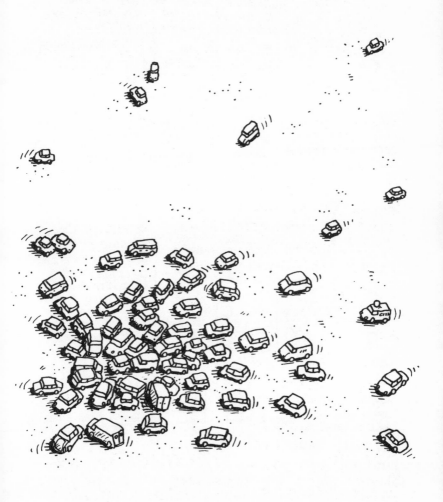

# T

**TRUTH** — One of the elemental forces which keep society functioning. Here we see how it works.

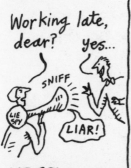

Working late, dear? yes...

SNIFF

LIE SPY

LIAR!

**LIE SPY** ANALYSES BODY ODOUR AND DECIDES WITHIN 3 SECONDS IF A LIE IS BEING TOLD.

## LIE GUARD

NEUTRALISES ODOUR EMISSIONS AND REPLACES THEM WITH THE SMELL OF TRUTH.

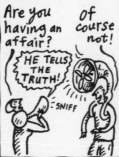

Are you having an affair?

Of course not!

HE TELLS THE TRUTH!

SNIFF

## LIE SPY SUPER

IGNORES TRUTH SMELL & READS SHIFTY EYE MOVEMENT INSTEAD.

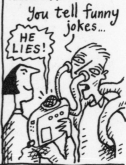

You tell funny jokes...

HE LIES!

## LIE GUARD GOLD

CALLS OUT YOUR INNOCENCE PREVENTING THE NEED TO LIE.

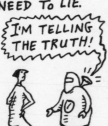

I'M TELLING THE TRUTH!

## LIE SPY ULTRA

DETECTS LIE SHIELDING DEVICES, PENETRATES THEM & SHOUTS ITS OPINION.

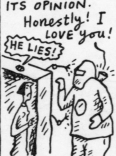

Honestly! I LOVE you!

HE LIES!

## LIE SPY BEHEMOTH & LIE GUARD ARMAGEDDON

WILL CARRY OUT DECEIT-FREE NEGOTIATIONS FOR THEIR OWNERS.

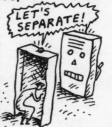

LET'S SEPARATE!

Is THIS BOOK telling you the truth? To find out, invest in APPLEBY's LIE SPY READER! Simply place the book, love letter, newspaper, etcetera, inside to get a quick answer.

# TUMMY NOISE ~

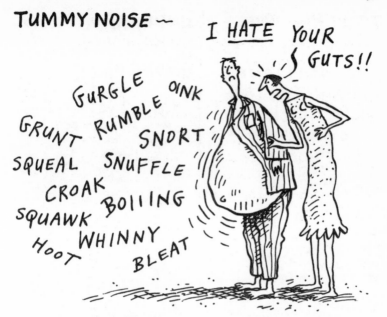

I HATE YOUR GUTS!!

GURGLE OINK
GRUNT RUMBLE SNORT
SQUEAL SNUFFLE
CROAK BOIIING
SQUAWK
HOOT WHINNY
BLEAT

# TURNING INTO A GIANT INSECT ~

UGH! Humans everywhere! SQUASH them!

SWAT them!

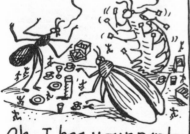

Oh. I beg your pardon. These REALLY ARE giant insects!

# TURNING INTO A TV ~

I can't help it!

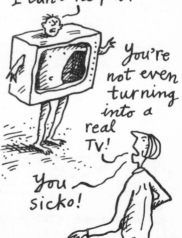

You're not even turning into a real TV!

You sicko!

# U

**UGLY** — See: ANUS.

**UNCLE** — See: FAMILY.

**UNCONDITIONAL LOVE** — What children think parents should give them.

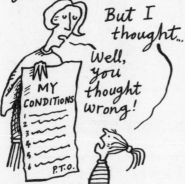

But I thought...

Well, you thought wrong!

MY CONDITIONS
1.
2.
3.
4.
5.
6.
P.T.O.

**UNCONSCIOUS** —

He's been unconscious ever since our marriage!

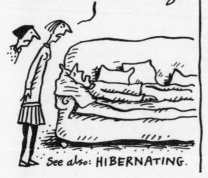

See also: HIBERNATING.

**UNDERARM** — A way of throwing a ball.

**UNDERFOOT** —

Ugh! I've stood in a pervert!

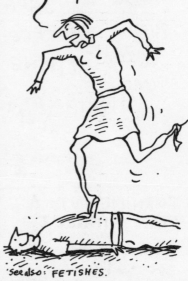

See also: FETISHES.

**UNDERWEAR** —

I'm wearing an overcoat as underwear!

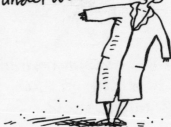

# UNDERMINE ~
Susan the secretary is being undermined by her friends and work colleagues.

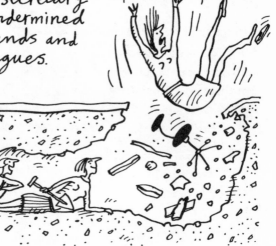

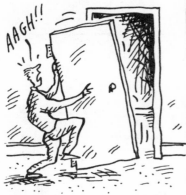

## UNHINGED ~

**AAGH!!**

UPSET ~ Caused by unrequited love and the biscuits running out.

## UNREQUITED LOVE ~

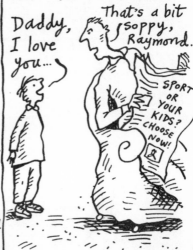

Daddy, I love you...

That's a bit soppy, Raymond.

SPORT OR YOUR KIDS? CHOOSE NOW!

See also: UNCONDITIONAL LOVE; LOVE.

# U

**UNPOPULAR** — Being unpopular will prevent you getting a swollen head, though it will also give you low self-esteem, bad body posture, depression and so on. Become popular by earning lots of money and buying some friends. In the meantime, console yourself by comparing yourself with the most unpopular man who ever lived.

HERE HE IS AS A BOY PLAYING CATCH WITH HIS FRIENDS:

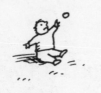

AND THIS IS HIM ON THE SCHOOL FOOTBALL TEAM:

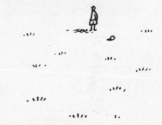

HERE HE IS AS AN ADULT OUT WALKING HIS DOG:

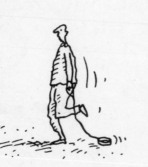

AND HERE HE IS MEETING ANOTHER UNPOPULAR PERSON:

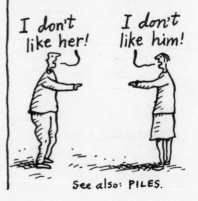

I don't like her!

I don't like him!

See also: PILES.

# UNUSUAL ATTRIBUTES~

**IF I HAD A SHAFT OF LIGHT SHINING OUT OF MY BOTTOM...**

**I'D USE IT TO HEAL THE SICK.**

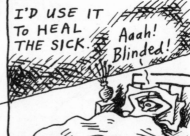

Aaah! Blinded!

**IT WOULD CUT DOWN MY ELECTRICITY BILL.**

**I'D POINT IT AT THE SKY TO SEE HOW FAR IT REACHED.**

**I'D BE ABLE TO WALK THE BABYSITTER HOME IN COMPLETE SAFETY.**

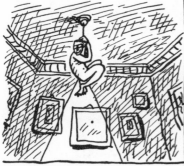

These backless pants are practical, modest and dignified

**I'D BE INSUFFERABLY SMUG ABOUT IT.**

I'm fabulous— and I can prove it. You see, the light shines out of my behind.

Well, I think you should see your GP.

# V

## VAIN –

I'm vain in vain, because I'm ugly!

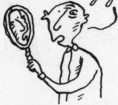

## VEGETABLE –
## VEGETARIAN –

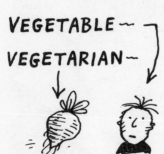

I may have mixed these two up.

## VENEREAL DISEASE
– A disease caught by having sex. These include: obsession, jealousy, embarrassment, depression, love and fear of having a small member

(applies to men only. Women get fear that <u>he's</u> got a small member.).

## VEST – Wear one.

## VIRGIN – A bit like chicken pox. When you're a virgin it seems to go on for ever, but when it's gone you're immune and can't catch it again.

I'm cured!

## VISIONS – Don't tell anyone if you have these. They won't understand.

## VOLUPTUOUSNESS –
Why are there no voluptuous men?

## WAIST —

Waste not, want not!

There's certainly no waist there!

"PROD"

## WARTS —

The following illustration, sketched from life, may prove shocking to my friend.

Amputation is the only course of action which will get rid of penis warts. Amputation of the warts, that is, not the entire organ. In most cases, anyway.

## WASPISH —

Ouch! You're being waspish today!

"STING!"

## WAXING —

Despite all the fuss about organic, natural food, I think waxing fruit is essential. I mean, who would buy hairy apples or lemons?

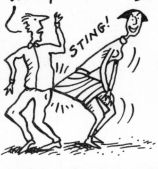

HAIRY LEMON →

## WET DREAM —

A dream in which you are having sex and someone throws a bucket of water over you. Dogs also have dreams like this.

# W

## WILD ANIMALS ~ Don't show any fear!

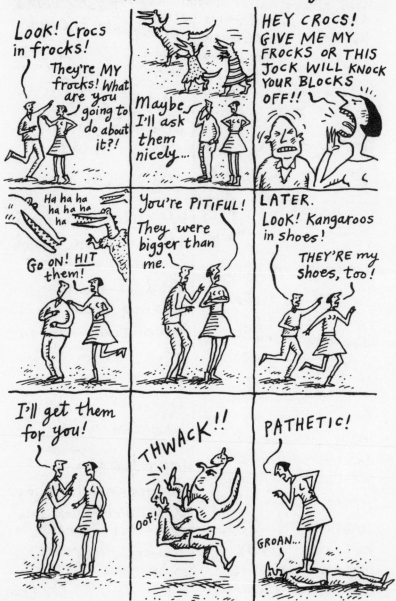

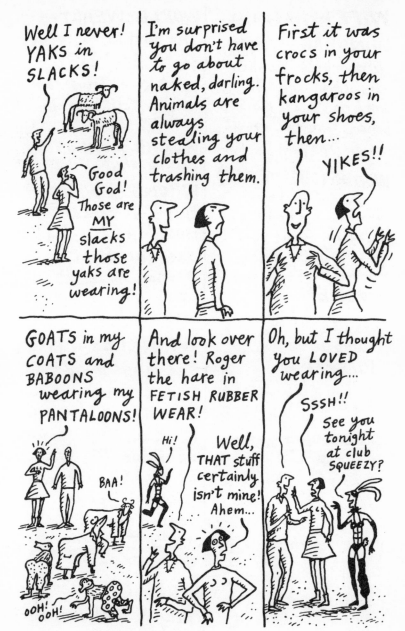

# W

**WIFE** ~ See FAMILY.

**WINDBAG** ~ A very humorous rubber cushion which makes fart noises when you sit on it. See also: FARTING.

**WOODS (OUT OF THE)** ~ Said a few moments before finding yourself in the frying pan.

**WOODEN** ~

You're a bit wooden, Pinocchio.

Look on the bright side. I never go flaccid.

**WORLD-WEARY** ~ The world is weary of us humans.

**WORK** ~ This can make you world-weary too.

**WORTHLESSNESS** ~ See: HUSBAND.

**WRONG** ~ What this book certainly isn't! And I shall sue the first person to say otherwise in a review!

**WRINKLES** ~ Like the rings inside a tree trunk, you can measure your age by counting your wrinkles. My friend is eighty-nine, while I remain only seventeen. Keep away from me with that axe!!

**WUB** ~ Character in a Philip K. Dick novel.

# X

**XIPHOID** ~ Sword-shaped. This is a really good word. See also: PENIS.

**X-RAY** ~ Sees right through you like your X-girlfriend or X-wife.

# Y

**YACHT** ~ This strange spelling proves that the Dutch are trying to take over the world.

**YOGA** ~ A vast catalogue of bizarre sexual positions masquerading as an exercise system. Here's one to try at your kitchen sink.

**YUCKY** ~ See: SEX.

# Z

**ZIPPER** ~ Good on clothes, better on animals.

**ZIT** ~ See: SPOTS.

**ZOMBIE** ~ The living dead. What I am as this book draws to a close at 3.00 am.

**ZYMURGY** ~ Branch of applied chemistry which deals with fermentation processes. It is the last word in any good encyclopedia, and means you can believe everything you just read.

171

# APPENDIX

Grit your teeth and take a deep breath. It's time to look at

# THE HUMAN BODY

# The HUMAN BODY

A catalogue of potential problems. Let's strip away the layers and see what's beneath.

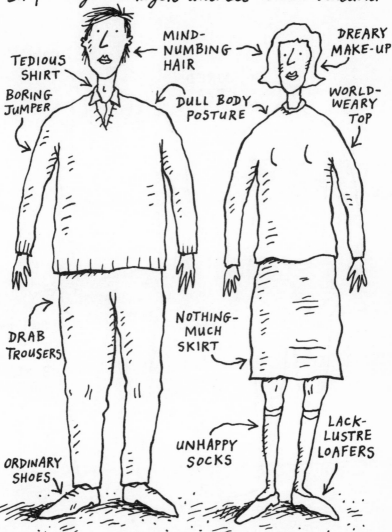

MIND-NUMBING HAIR

DREARY MAKE-UP

TEDIOUS SHIRT

BORING JUMPER

DULL BODY POSTURE

WORLD-WEARY TOP

DRAB TROUSERS

NOTHING-MUCH SKIRT

ORDINARY SHOES

UNHAPPY SOCKS

LACK-LUSTRE LOAFERS

DRESS SENSE - none.

# UNDERWEAR ~ Limp, non-matching and exhausted lingerie.

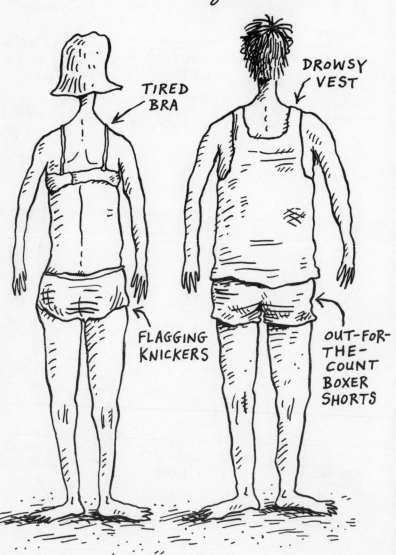

TIRED BRA

DROWSY VEST

FLAGGING KNICKERS

OUT-FOR-THE-COUNT BOXER SHORTS

# The NAKED BODY

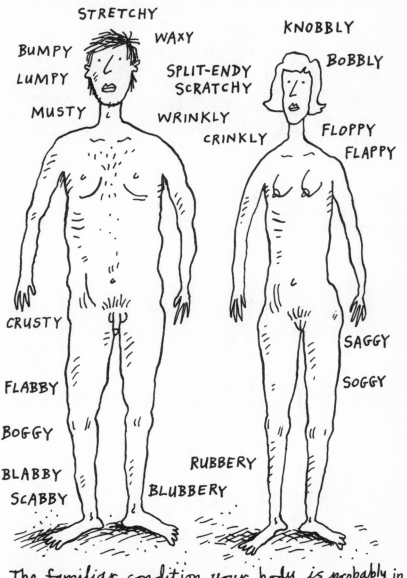

STRETCHY

BUMPY
LUMPY

MUSTY

WAXY

SPLIT-ENDY
SCRATCHY

WRINKLY
CRINKLY

KNOBBLY

BOBBLY

FLOPPY
FLAPPY

CRUSTY

FLABBY

BOGGY

BLABBY
SCABBY

RUBBERY
BLUBBERY

SAGGY

SOGGY

The familiar condition your body is probably in.

# The DISCHARGING BODY

Unpleasant I know, but it must be faced.

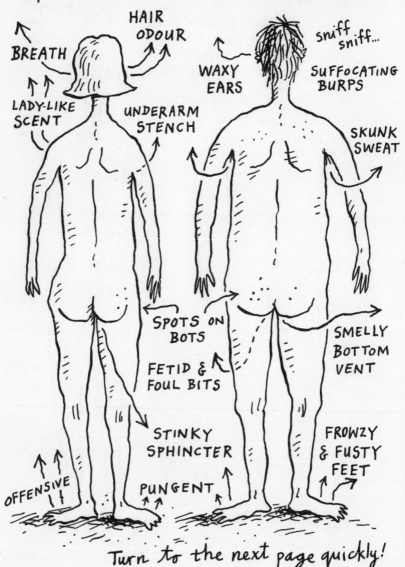

BREATH

HAIR ODOUR

LADY-LIKE SCENT

UNDERARM STENCH

WAXY EARS

sniff sniff...

SUFFOCATING BURPS

SKUNK SWEAT

SPOTS ON BOTS

FETID & FOUL BITS

SMELLY BOTTOM VENT

STINKY SPHINCTER

PUNGENT

OFFENSIVE

FROWZY & FUSTY FEET

Turn to the next page quickly!

# The MUSCLES

They look rather like spaghetti, don't they, and without exercise that is how they end up - soggy and floppy.

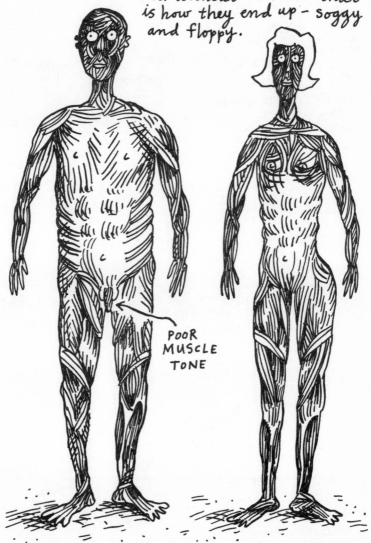

POOR
MUSCLE
TONE

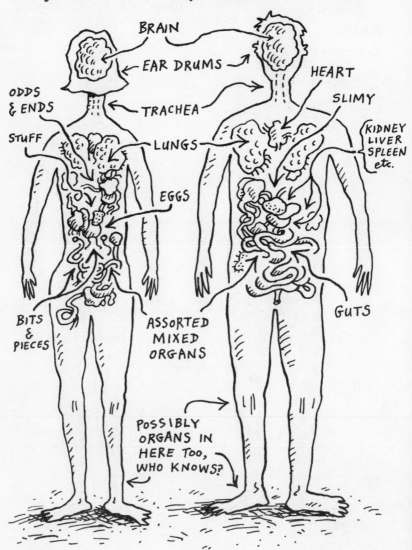

# The SKELETON

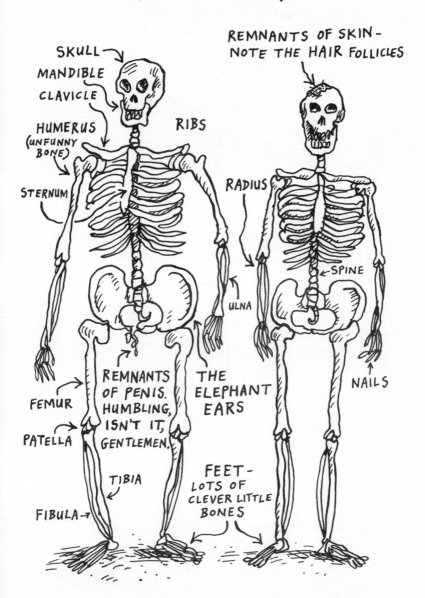

SKULL

MANDIBLE

CLAVICLE

HUMERUS
(UNFUNNY
BONE)

STERNUM

RIBS

RADIUS

ULNA

SPINE

REMNANTS OF SKIN-
NOTE THE HAIR FOLLICLES

NAILS

REMNANTS
OF PENIS.
HUMBLING,
ISN'T IT,
GENTLEMEN.

THE
ELEPHANT
EARS

FEMUR

PATELLA

TIBIA

FIBULA →

FEET-
LOTS OF
CLEVER LITTLE
BONES

HERE ARE two splendid carriages in which to journey to the next world.

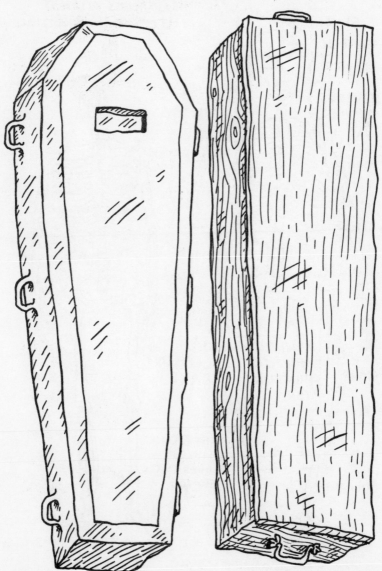

PLASTIC WITH SNAP-ON LIDS & WOOD-EFFECT FINISH

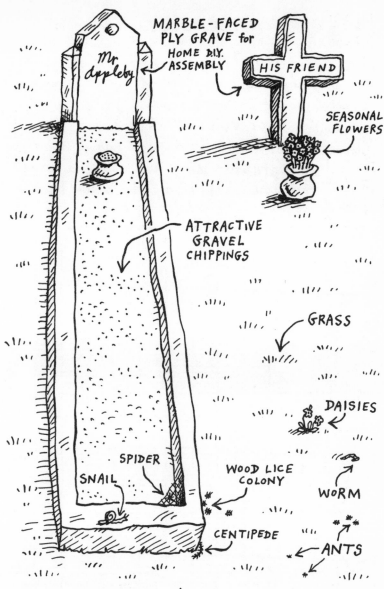

MARBLE-FACED PLY GRAVE for HOME D.I.Y. ASSEMBLY

Mr Appleby

HIS FRIEND

SEASONAL FLOWERS

ATTRACTIVE GRAVEL CHIPPINGS

GRASS

DAISIES

SPIDER

SNAIL

WOOD LICE COLONY

WORM

CENTIPEDE

ANTS

So life goes on... though not for me and you, of course.

183

# CHECKLIST

How are you doing? Keep track of your ups and downs by plotting your weekly progress on the chart below. Judge your problem's improvement on a scale of 1 (almost gone) to 10 (rampant) and mark it on the graph. Why not make a huge chart for your kitchen? It will be a great topic of conversation!

| MY PROBLEM | WEEK 1 | WEEK 2 | WEEK 3 | WEEK 4 | WEEK 5 | WEEK 6 | WEEK 7 | WEEK 8 | WEEK 9 | WEEK 10 |
|---|---|---|---|---|---|---|---|---|---|---|
|  |  |  |  |  |  |  |  |  |  |  |
|  |  |  |  |  |  |  |  |  |  |  |
|  |  |  |  |  |  |  |  |  |  |  |
|  |  |  |  |  |  |  |  |  |  |  |
|  |  |  |  |  |  |  |  |  |  |  |

# NOTES

# ABOUT THE AUTHOR

STEVEN APPLEBY *is twenty-nine, or fourty-four. He may even be fifty-six. If not yet, then one day.*

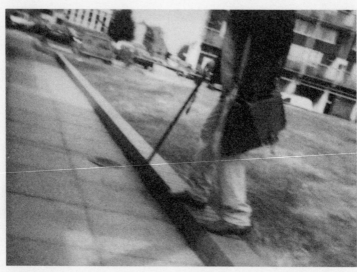

PHOTO BY: JASPER APPLEBY SHERRING

A rare photograph of the author wearing clothes. Or it may be his friend.

Other life-enhancing books by STEVEN APPLEBY which you may find useful include:

NORMAL SEX

MEN – THE TRUTH!

MISERABLE/HAPPY FAMILIES

THE SECRET THOUGHTS OF:
  MEN/ WOMEN/ DOGS
  CATS/ BABIES/ YOURSELF

ANTMEN CARRY AWAY MY
  THOUGHTS AS SOON AS
  I THINK THEM

ALIEN INVASION! THE COMPLETE
  GUIDE TO HAVING CHILDREN

THE TRUTH ABOUT LOVE

# AFTERWORD

The pace of change in our modern world is now so fast that since you began reading this book it has become out of date. The publishers suggest that you should discard this old copy and purchase a new, fresh, up-to-the-minute one from your local bookstore or at their website —
www.bloomsbury.com

If Steven Appleby had a website it would be —
www.stevenappleby.com

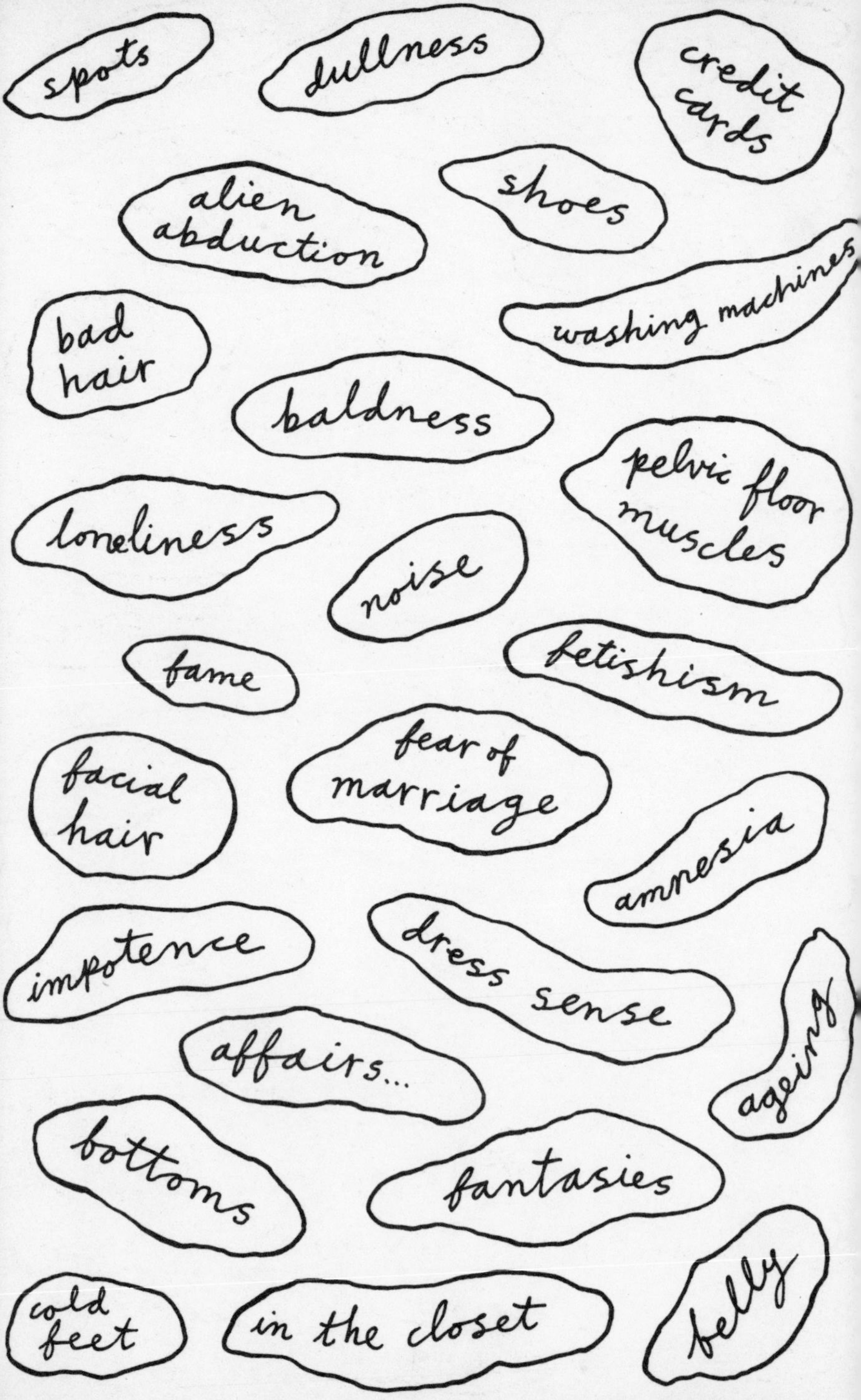

spots

dullness

credit cards

alien abduction

shoes

washing machines

bad hair

baldness

pelvic floor muscles

loneliness

noise

fame

fetishism

facial hair

fear of marriage

amnesia

impotence

dress sense

affairs...

ageing

bottoms

fantasies

cold feet

in the closet

belly